MUSCULAR POWER AND BEAUTY

Containing Detailed Instructions for the Development of the External Muscular System to its Utmost Degree of Perfection

BY

BERNARR MACFADDEN

Fredonia Books
Amsterdam, The Netherlands

Muscular Power and Beauty

by
Bernarr Macfadden

ISBN: 1-58963-513-2

Reprinted from the 1906 edition

Fredonia Books
Amsterdam, The Netherlands
http://www.fredoniabooks.com

CONTENTS

3

CONTENTS

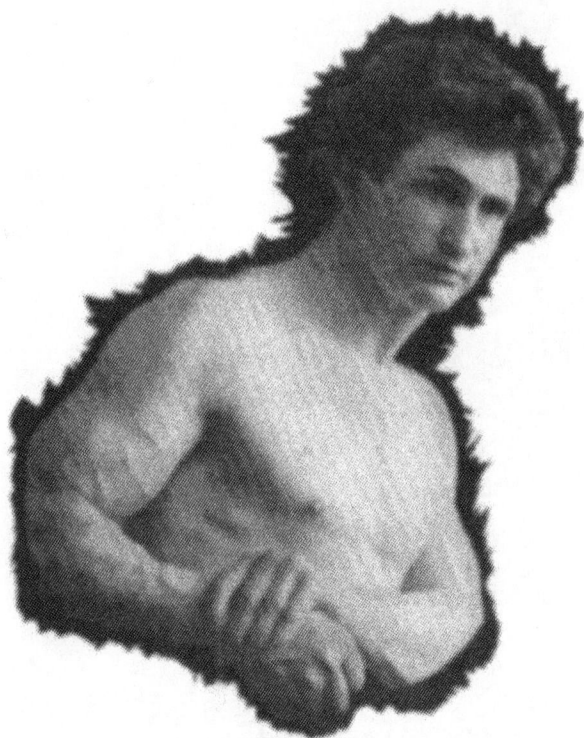

Bernarr Macfadden

PREFACE

Muscular power is beginning to assume its proper importance in the minds of every sensible man and woman. A few years ago, so-called refined persons were inclined to belittle its value. They affected to associate large, well-developed muscles with various undesirable mental and bodily characteristics. But the physical culture movement has wrought a marvelous change in these as in others. As true manhood and womanhood are founded upon strong, beautifully developed physiques, these last are being accorded the recognition which they deserve. You cannot exaggerate the value of muscular power and beauty. In erecting a building, the material that enters into its construction is of the utmost importance. How much more important then is it that that used in the construction of the human body is of he soundest? By which is more particularly meant, strong, symmetrically formed muscles. For a sound muscular system in nearly every case, means the possession of equal strength in your functional organism. It also insures the nervous vigor that is so essential in the attaining of one's objects of life, no matter whether physical or mental energy is required.

The exercises presented in this book furnish about the most effective method of developing the muscular system, that can be secured outside of the gymnasium or from the use of elaborate apparatus. I have received hundreds of letters from those who have used the exercises to great advantage. Also has there been a great demand for a book of instructions that would supply detailed information for developing defective parts of the body, and for bringing about the highest degree of strength and symmetrical outlines in all parts of the physical system. As will be noted, a special chapter is devoted to the exercises applicable to each of the important groups of muscles. If there is a muscular defect of any kind, one can readily turn to the chapter giving instructions for developing the muscles that are thus lacking in symmetry and strength. The proper use of weak muscles will in every case remedy their deficiencies with surprising rapidity. Apart from this, however, I think that in this book will be found information that will be of great value to everyone striving for physical improvement. That it may furnish the encouragement and yield the instruction necessary to the building of beautiful human bodies, is the wish of the author.

Bernarr Macfadden

MUSCULAR POWER AND BEAUTY

CHAPTER I.

The Perfect Man! What a picture of health, of power, of noble beauty these words conjure up before our mental vision! For we of to-day are becoming re-born in the wisdom of the ancients in that we no longer see anything but the pitiful or contemptible in the physique that is not strong, undefiled and wholesome.

Physically blemished or undeveloped manhood would always arouse disgust in us did we not sometimes pity the unhappy one so afflicted. And when the blemish exists without need—as it does in nearly all cases—we wonder whether it is due to ignorance, to indifference or self-complacency. Why any man will be puny when he may as easily be powerful, why he will wilfully deny himself any charm of grace or of beauty when these last can be readily secured—these are problems that are most perplexing to us.

The men of ancient Greece and Rome were—MEN! Men powerful in every attribute of mind and of body, men able to dare and to do, men whose feet trod in conquest and whose war-banners waved victorious in every portion of the then known world; men made restless by the lust of travel, men of parts in the arts and in statecraft! Civilization can reach no stage so

13

perfect that it will not turn gratefully back to Greece and to Rome to contemplate those noble conceptions of the best in the life of the mind and of the body that the ancients have dowered to us for all time.

Through the centuries, our universities have handed down to us the fruits of the mental conquests of these two grand and virile races of old. And now, tardily enough to be sure, we are turning back to these same great races for our strongest and truest ideals of physical manhood.

Magnificently perfect do the men of old stand out before us! We have reliable records of them as they were. They were strong and beautiful men, and through their literature we know all of that which made them so. We possess a perfect impression of the classic type, and we know the secret of its composition. What the Greeks and the Romans were, we can become also; aye, we can surpass them, for we possess greater and more exact knowledge of the intricate machinery of the body, and we know better how to care for and train that body.

Strength and beauty were deified in Greece and in Rome.. Greek mythology became in turn the property of the Romans. In this mythology we find the aspirations of the people strongly outlined. We realize how they yearned for strength and for the beauty that is a part of it. History tells us how truly great these people were as long as they remained faithful to their ideals. History also tells us how the possession of wealth and the luxury that followed in its train destroyed these aspirations after manliness, and how in turn each of the two great states fell in consequence. We of to-day are citizens of the richest and greatest of nations. Let us profit by the lessons of history. Ere it is too late,

let us go back to the glorious old standards of what the
Perfect Man was and must be and our national efficacy
and potency will be preserved for all time.

The gods and goddesses of the Greeks and Romans
were originally embodiments of the national ideals.
They were strong, agile, virile. Apollo, Hercules, Juno,
Venus, Diana—all without physical blemish! The
departures from morality which legend attributes
to some of them, were not identified with them until
a luxury debased people corrupted what was an initially
pure mythology. Apollo and Hercules were favorite
sons of Zeus or Jupiter, and they stand for the two
types of men of whom we have the most need to-day.

Apollo was the most glorious and beautiful of the
gods, the representative of life and light; he was lithe
and supple, skilled in the chase, and terrible in combat
with man or beast. Yet he was versed in all the Arts
and became the leader of the Muses. He was the ideal
of what the brainy leader of men and of women should
be.

Statues handed down to us by the ancients show the
strength and beauty of this young god as conceived by
them. His face is instinct with majesty, in which there
is, withal, a cheerful serenity of temper. He is shown
with fair, clustering locks surmounting a head perfect
in its proportions, and every line of his contour is truly
and wonderfully beautiful. Such statues are the reali-
zations in marble of the spirit and genius of the ancients.

Leto was Apollo's mother. Tradition relates that,
forced, through the jealousy of Juno, to wander during
her pregnancy, Leto led the outdoor life. And so she
learned to draw her health from Nature's heaving
bosom and absorb all that was best and noblest in her
teacher. Living simply, therefore, and amid inanimate

grandeur, Leto's was an ideal pregnancy, and the fruit thereof was seen in her god-like son.

Apollo was indeed that which such pre-natal influences might be expected to produce. He was beloved by his worshippers, he carried his leadership by sheer might of both mind and body. It is true that he had the misfortune to be the father of Esculapius, the founder of the practice of medicine, but there is likely to be one disappointing son in all families. And as Apollo led men, so we find that his attributes made him a leader on the heights of Olympus.

In Hercules we have a type, not of the intellectual guide, but of the man of deeds, the brawny, powerful laborer. The twelve prodigious tasks of Hercules, all of which he performed successfully, are indicative of the best results of sturdy manual toil and untiring industry. Hercules is pictured to us as possessing an altogether different sort of physical perfection from that of his intellectual brother; for Hercules had a smaller head, a short, bull-like neck, and a body that was massive instead of lithe and supple. Yet he was credited with many kindly and helpful traits; he was ever ready to place his great strength at the service of those who needed it. It followed, as a matter of course, that he lived out of doors and was ever watchful for opportunities to develop his strength.

It may not be out of place to note that the end of Hercules' earthly career came through drugs. Deianira, tortured by jealousy, sent him a present of a sacrificial robe that had been anointed with a poisonous ointment. Hercules assumed this robe and went before an altar. The poisons in the ointment penetrated his body, causing such unconquerable anguish that the hero built himself a funeral pyre and lighting it, lay upon it until he was consumed.   But his apotheosis followed and men worshipped him for his great strength and his helpfulness to others.

And today we find that while the worship of strength and of all phases of manly beauty is less idolatrous, yet it is none the less general and sincere.   The classic ideal of powerful and prepossessing manhood once more obtains.   And we have a type of such manhood that is new in our day, one that is popularly designated as the "college man."   He might with more truth be styled the Physical Culture Man.   In him we see again reproduced the god-like ideal of the ancients.   Wherever we find this superb specimen of young manhood, erect, powerful, square-shouldered, with jaw firmly set, having eyes clear, kindly and sparkling, and face radiant with health and intelligence—all of us must admire if not envy him.   But he is merely the sample of what all men may become who follow and practice the laws of the physical culture life.

Power and beauty are not for the favored few; they may become the property of any man in normal health who thinks their possession worth an expenditure of effort.   It is the mission of this volume to point the way to the acquisition of these attributes plainly and unerringly, and in such terms that "he who runs may read" and that to his lasting advantage.

CHAPTER II.

Apollo, rather than Hercules, stands for the type of
physical manhood that is demanded to-day. Powerful
muscular development there must be in the ideal man,
but there must also be a counterpoise of grace and of
intellect.

, True muscular development not only increases
the general functional powers; but works marvellous
effects upon those vigilant servants of the brain, the
nerves, which are the master organs of the body.
Muscular development brings in its train virile qualities
to the blood, and this blood nourishes all the tissues
of the body, including, of course, those of the brain.
In other words, the more a man exercises his muscles—
always within reason—the purer and better vitalized
his blood becomes. And the better the blood, the
purer and more enduring will be every tissue in his

18

body; as has just been said, such blood feeds even the brain itself.

But the question will very naturally arise: What is the best system of bodily training to be followed? In this volume I shall answer the question by presenting fully and faithfully the system that my own hard-earned experience has shown me to be the best and the quickest method of attaining the highest muscular ideal.

The ancient Greeks, and likewise the Romans, were content with the simplest of accessories. The perfect man was developed without the aid of any costly gymnastic accessories. The youth of ancient days found full scope for his powers in swimming, running, leaping, wrestling, throwing the discus, riding and in bouts with arms.

With the resurrection of the Greek and Roman ideals of manliness we find a rather strange departure from ancient methods. Archibald Maclaren, who originated the present system of gymnastics at Oxford University, and who may be regarded as the father of modern physical training in England and in this country, introduced a scheme for the employment of numerous, ponderous and rather costly "machines." With the most careful economy it would require an outlay of many hundreds of dollars to fit up a small gymnasium with the different kinds of apparatus that the genius of Maclaren has bequeathed to us. Valuable these machines doubtless are in the creation of powerful muscles, yet they are also unnecessary. Just as perfect muscular conditions can be brought about without the aid of the Maclaren machines, and that, too, with more speedy results.

We are most of us familiar with the devices of

Maclaren, for they are on exhibition in nearly every American gymnasium. There are the horizontal and parallel bars, the flying rings, the trapeze, the ladders, the elastic ladders, the rings in series, the bridge ladders, the planks with and without footholds, the "prepared wall," the vertical ropes, the beam and all the bewildering what-nots of the gymnasium. American genius has added the wall-machines with weights. The use of these devices, and in addition, foot-ball, baseball, rowing and field and track athletics in general, make up the system that has come to us mainly through the efforts of Maclaren and his co-workers.

Now, my friends, all this gymnastic apparatus is as unnecessary as it is costly. Mind you, I do not wish to be understood in the least as discrediting the splendid missionary work of Maclaren and all those who have followed in his footsteps. If you have free access to a gymnasium, all of the work that is done there,—if you employ it in connection with your own good common sense and do not overtrain—will result to your benefit. If you have not access to a gymnasium, however, and do not feel like expending the money for costly accessories, you will save a good deal of hard-earned money by following in every detail the course that I shall outline. In any case you will soon discover, as I have done, that the methods offered in this volume are of infinitely greater value in the building up of the best muscular conditions obtainable than are those of the gymnasium.

So far it has been to our university gymnasiums that we have turned for our ideas of how to build the perfect body. Certainly these college gymnasia, with their complicated devices and their vast amount of hard physical work, have produced good results. But

the tendency has already set in strongly toward lighter
and still lighter work, and with less and less inanimate
apparatus.

Take the methods of physical instruction, for
instance, that are now in vogue at the Military Academy
at West Point, and at the Naval Academy at Annapolis·
The cadets who graduate from these two great Ameri
can institutions average as fine a display of physical
manhood as could be desired.   The almost inexhausti-
ble purse of Uncle Sam is opened freely in the equip-
ment of the gymnasia at these places.   Yet for years
the gradual discarding of heavy, inanimate apparatus
has been going on.   And though the preference for
lighter work and the gradual abolition of much of the
machine-work were severely criticized at first, the
results have justified the changes.   The graduates of
to-day make a better average showing than those of
former years.

So the ice has been broken.   To-day, those who are
interested in the best possible development of the
human body are prepared to take up a course of training as simple as was that of the ancient Greeks and
Romans.   Years and years ago I became convinced of
the need of discarding heavy and costly apparatus in
favor of "devices" that are supplied in the main to man
by his own body.   The few extraneous articles that are
needed, are such as are constantly at hand, or may be
made quickly through the exercise of a little ordinary
ingenuity and handicraft.

And while studying almost incessantly along these
lines of exercises that more closely approximate the
methods of the ancient athletes, I have not failed to
note the results as compared with those obtained in the
ordinary gymnasium.   The new methods are incom-

parably better than those in vogue during the last few decades. The new methods are closely in touch with those that made manly strength and beauty the rule rather than the exception in classic periods. And these new methods have the incalculably great advantage of being wholly in accord with our modern knowledge of anatomy, physiology and all the complexities of the body's varied functions and needs. This knowledge was denied the ancients, whose system of training, simple and effective as it was, was based, as Maclaren has pointed out, on observation of effects and not on knowledge of causes.

These latest discoveries as to the quickest, surest and at the same time simplest methods of attaining the highest physical ideals of perfect manhood and surpassing womanhood are now offered in their entirety for the first time. The task of arranging this complete system of exercises has been long and laborious. But the results and amazing benefits have been noted so carefully and methodically, that I can guarantee that the exercises comprise the best system of physical training that has yet been devised for the development of humanity on the lines of bodily perfection.

CHAPTER III.

Developing Great Lung Capacity is of the Highest Importance in the Attainment of Unusual Muscular Power.

"The maintenance of animal life necessitates the continual absorption of oxygen and excretion of carbonic acid . . . . . the blood being the medium by which these gases are carried."—Kirkes.

To the intelligent trainer of the human body it is amazing that any one should attempt to reach great muscular development without paying the utmost heed to increasing the capacity of the lungs. Yet this is what thousands and thousands of men and women are attempting every day. Go into any gymnasium, or into any school where the instructor is not intelligent and alert, and you will see just what I mean.

In such institutions we may note young men working like beavers to pile on muscle and yet more muscle, hard muscle and still tougher muscle. But watch them when they cease work for a few moments. Note whether they are stoop-shouldered. Look to see if their shoulder-points droop forward, contracting and narrowing the chest. Observe whether they are breathing deeply and *properly,* or whether they take their breath in short, choppy gasps, and relax even this form of deep breathing as soon as their panting for air is over.

Would-be athletes who treat their lungs in this fashion are denying themselves the very benefits that they profess to seek. Men who do not at all times, when in the quest for powerful muscles, keep their minds constantly on the subject of the most perfect development of lung capacity, are stultifying their work and nullifying their efforts.

You cannot become extremely muscular, in the real sense of the word, unless your lung capacity is pushed to the utmost limit of normal development! You might as well try to satisfy hunger with nothing but water.

Muscle-making is accomplished by breaking down the individual cells of which every tissue in the body— whether of bone or of flesh—is composed. As these tiny cells are broken down, new ones take their place; and when the old and useless cells are destroyed through vigorous exercise, the new cells that take their places are larger, more vigorous *and more numerous.* Each one of these little cells, of microscopic size, is a tiny but complete living body by itself. Like all other living bodies it has the power of reproducing itself. Before the old cell dies it gives birth to a new one. If the old cell has been a healthy one, full of vim and vigor, its offspring are more numerous; the old cell gives birth to two or more new ones before it is destroyed. It is in this way that exercise, while eliminating the old cell, produces in its place more numerous cells of added v gor and vitality.

Now, the material that is used for the building up of these new cells, and thereby for the building up of newer and better tissues al through the body, is taken from the food that is digested in the stomach and in the small intestine. This vitalized nourishment is carried to all parts of the body by the blood on its mission of building up the new cells, and hence the tissues.

But what of the dead matter—the portions of the old cells that are constantly dying off? Such matter must be removed from the body, or very soon the system will become so clogged that death will follow from stagnation or toxic conditions Not only does the blood carry new matter to build up the cells and tissue; but it is the blood that must bring the dead matter back to the lungs and the excreting organs, to be by them cast out of the body.

The dead matter is found in the tissues mainly in the form of carbon and its compounds. The new blood that the arteries carry from the heart to every portion of the body is laden with oxygen from the air that we breathe. The carbon is burned up by, or rather combines with, the oxygen and the result is a new compound, a gas that is called carbonic acid gas, or carbon dioxide. By the time that the bright red arterial blood has performed its mission of carrying new cell-food to the tissues, and has become the dark-colored, impure venous blood, it is heavily charged with the carbonic acid gas and other products of the burning up of the carbon by the oxygen.

The kidneys, the liver, the skin, and the large intestine do their share of the work of excreting waste matter from the body—*but of this same work the lungs form the great central market wherein is effected the exchange of the bulk of the worthless waste matter for the new and good matter that is used in building and strengthening and invigorating the physical system.*

These lungs of ours fill the greater portion of that part of the body which is called the chest or thorax. The size of the lungs alone ought to indicate their wonderful importance. On a superficial examination of a pair of lungs you would see, apparently, two masses of spongy material with several tubes or passages running through them. As a matter of fact a close examination, aided by a microscope, would show that the lungs, so far from being spongy masses, are two great organs that are made up of networks of infinitely fine air passages and tiny blood vessels.

If we consider the respiratory organs we shall find, beginning with the throat, first, the trachea, or windpipe. This trachea divides into two smaller air passages that are called the bronchi. One bronchus passes into the right lung, and the other into the left. Each bronchus is in turn subdivided, and these subdivisions are again subdivided, and so on and on, each new subdivision becoming smaller and smaller as the division continues. At the extreme ends of the very smallest air passages are the alveolar cells, or air-cells. Thus through this network of air-passages the inhaled air is carried to every one of the tiniest nooks and crevices of the lungs.

From the right side of the heart the impure venous blood, laden with the carbonic acid gas and foulness that result from the destruction of the old, dead cells, flows into the lungs. This impure blood passes through divisions and subdivisions of the larger blood vessels until, in the tinier blood vessels, the impure blood is brought into contact with the air that is being poured out through the countless alveolar cells. Only the thinnest kind of membranes separate the impure venous blood and the new, pure air that has just been inhaled by the lungs. These membranes permit of the passage of the carbonic acid gas and foul moisture into the air passages, and permit also the passage of the

new, fresh oxygen from the outer air into the blood
that has just been relieved of its impurities.

An inhalation of air supplies the new oxygen that the
purified b ood needs before it can start properly
equipped on its new round through the body; while
the act of exhaling air from the lungs forces out of the
body all of the poisonous gas that the venous blood
had brought to the lungs. It is evident, therefore,
that if the work of building up the body and of remov-
ing the waste, dead cell-matter is to be carried on without hindrance or delay, the supplies of fresh air to the
blood must be both frequent and generous. *Our
vitality depends absolutely upon the quantity of air that
we breathe into the lungs!*

The lungs, my readers, cannot hold any more air
than their capacity permits. If you have failed, so
far, to develop splendid lung capacity, then you have
wilfully or ignorantly failed to provide one of the
principal means by which the building of a mc e
powerful body is alone possible. Make a note of
this, think it over again and again, and never forget it!

How is this great and indispensable lung capacity to
be obtained? In a very simple way. By taking in
great, deep breaths of air, filling your lungs to the
utmost of their apparent capacity, and by exercises
that will aid in throwing out the ribs and expanding
the chest. Any plan that throws out the chest, either
deep breathing or muscular exercise, or what not, will
aid in increasing your lung capacity. Between the
ribs are cartilages that hold the former in place and
serve as cushions between them. Every time that the
ribs are thrown upward and forward, the cartilages are
made to stretch. Enough of this stretching makes the

cartilages longer and more elastic. As time goes on, the ribs can be made to move further forward and upward at each inspiration of air. This constant exercise, too, strengthens the chest muscles, and they in consequence are able to lift the ribs more easily.

Now, as the ribs go forward and upward, our lungs follow, for they are very elastic. They are so elastic, in fact, that they would naturally contract away from the walls formed by the ribs, were it not for the pressure of the inhaled air against the *inner* surfaces of their air passages. Whenever the chest muscles become strong enough to lift the ribs further and further upward and outward, and the exercised and stretched cartilages between the ribs permit of the movement, the cavity of the chest is enlarged. When this enlargement takes place, the lungs follow the rib-walls, and thus the lungs themselves become more and more expanded. This greater lung capacity makes it possible to inhale more and yet more air. The changes in the bodily tissues can therefore go on more rapidly, and the carbonic acid gas and the foul moisture are more quickly and thoroughly removed from the blood. This leaves the blood in a proper condition to do its work of carrying nourishment to the cells and tissues. And it follows that a larger and better body is built up in the place of the old body. The muscles become larger, harder, firmer, more powerful, vitality is increased, health is perfected and the man is born again, so to speak!

Read this over and over again if needs be, my friend. Don't let one iota of this information as to the prime importance of great lung power as a foundation for great muscular strength, escape you.   Don't make the silly mistake of neglecting to develop your lung capacity to its very utmost when you are trying to obtain muscles, if not of Herculean, yet of satisfactory dimensions.

CHAPTER IV.

EXERCISES FOR DEVELOPING THE LUNGS.

"Under the conditions of a sedentary life, nearly one-half of the air cells in the lungs remain habitually contracted, and take scarcely any part in the act of respiration. These cells thus lose their elasticity, the chest itself becomes narrow and shrunken, and when a sudden call is made for a full and deep inspiration, the lungs cannot respond satisfactorily."—H. RIPPON SEYMOUR.

In addition to the reasons that I offered in the last chapter as to why great lung capacity must be provided for, we find another and very excellent reason in the statement of the author quoted above. He who has not the best kind of lung expansion is incapable of taking the sudden deep, full breaths that are absolutely needed when any unusual muscular exertion is to be made.

As to the kinds of exercises that one must take in order to put the lungs in their best possible condition, it will be seen that Nature is always logical in her demands. Since we need larger chest dimensions in order that we may breathe as deeply as severe muscular exertion demands, it is necessary that we exercise the muscles that must be employed in the work of thus breathing. And we exercise those muscles by forcing them to perform, to the best of their ability, the kind of work that we want them to do.

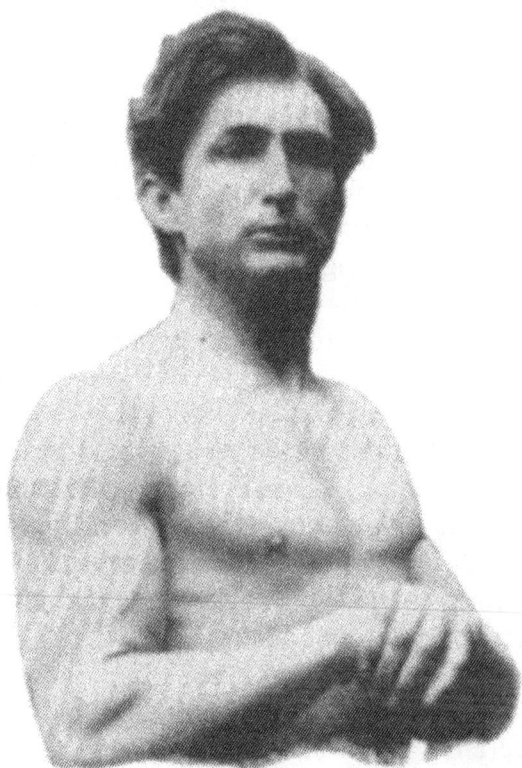

Photograph No. 1.

Exercise No. 1. Form the mouth so that there will be a very small opening; then draw in the breath very slowly yet forcibly until the abdominal regions and chest have been filled to their fullest capacity. If desired you can draw the air through a small pipe stem or breathing tube when taking this exercise, or you can close the nostrils partially with the fingers and draw in the air slowly through the nostrils. This exercise greatly strengthens the muscles used while drawing in the breath.

Remember that the two exercises that I advise for the enlarging of lung capacity are the basis, the foundation-work of all great muscular development!

Exercise number one, as shown in photograph number one, explains the method of inhaling air. The descriptive text should be read very carefully; and should be followed in the work with equal care. Do not breathe hurriedly. Do not try to see how quickly you can get the lungs filled. Take the inspiration slowly, and inhale the breath regularly right throughout the work. Do not stop inhaling until you feel that your lungs have been filled to the very last notch of capacity.

As soon as you gotten the idea of this fully, you are ready for the complemental exercise that is illustrated in photograph number two. In this, the work is exactly opposite. Now, you exhale a breath by a reversal of the process that you used in drawing in air. And this work should be done just as slowly and as regularly as in the case of the first exercise.

From the outset, and no matter how long you have been practicing these two exercises, you should begin every bout of exercise with several repetitions of each of these breathing movements. Practice them between any two other feats of exercise. Do so when you are resting, and be sure to breathe as deeply and fully as you can during any kind of muscular exercise. Get into the habit of practicing these two exercises at frequent intervals through the day, whether you are resting, or engaged in your usual occupations. Take these exercises in the morning, as soon as you are out of bed. Go through them at night, just before you get into bed. Whenever possible take them in the open air. There is more and purer oxygen out-of-doors

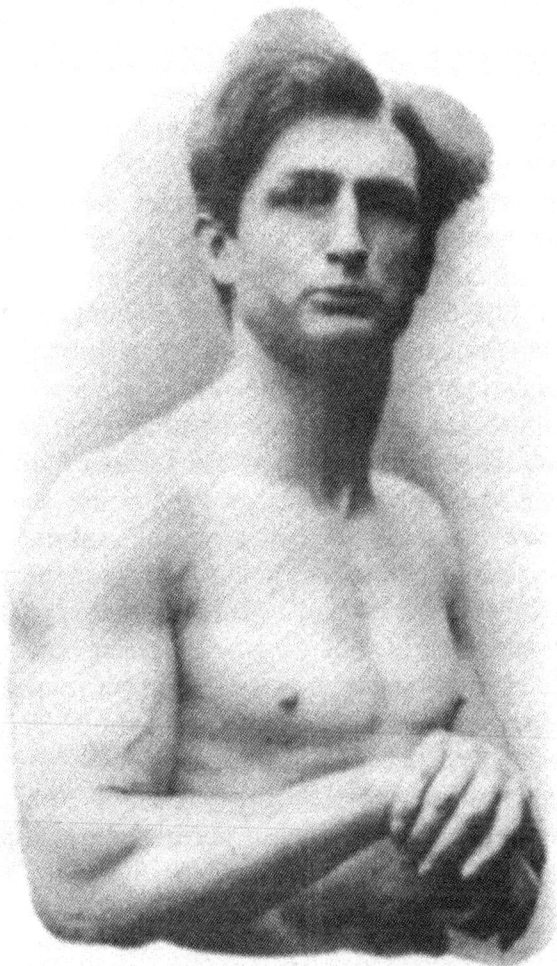

Photograph No. 2.

Exercise No. 2. This is a similar exercise to the preceding, though the force is exerted while expelling the breath instead of while inhaling it. First fill your lungs completely, then forming the mouth into a small opening, as described before, force the air out very slowly yet vigorously. A pipe stem or breathing tube can be used through which to force the air in this as in the preceding exercise if you desire, or it can be taken while partially closing the nostrils with the fingers. This exercise is for strengthening the expelling muscles of the chest used in breathing.

than there can be in any wall-enclosed room, no matter how well ventilated the latter.

Many readers are sure to wonder why these two exercises need to be gone through so slowly, with the mouth but little open. Why could not the exercise be taken just as well with the mouth wide open? The reason is, that when you breathe in slowly through a very small opening of the mouth you keep the chest muscles and inter-rib cartilages that are set in motion longer at their work. You subject these muscles and cartilages to a species of strain that is not too severe. You make them do steady, gradual, sustained work, and it is this sort of work that strengthens the muscles and cartilages more than rapid work continued for a shorter time could do. With constant and patient repetition of these exercises, the chest muscles will become rapidly stronger, the cartilages more elastic, and the frequent use of the tape measure will show you that your capacity for lung expansion is increasing.

It is wonderful work, this building up of the lungs! It is work that is likely to add many years and incalculable health and happiness to your life.

CHAPTER V.

Anatomical Structure of the Chest Muscles.

Very closely allied to the development of the lungs is the development of the chest muscles. Yet it is not alone for breathing power that the chest muscles must be improved. Such muscles are of great use in other processes than breathing. The pectoral muscles, for instance, figure in a variety of movements of the arms and shoulders. To develop the biceps, therefore, at the expense of the pectorals would be but to half develop the arms.

Besides the pectorals, of which I shall say more later, the important muscles of the chest are the intercostals and the serratus magnus. (Now do not be dismayed at these Latin names. They are the names used by the anatomists, and I shall make the uses of these muscles quite plain to you.)

The intercostals are the muscles mentioned in the preceding chapter: They lie between the ribs, much on the same plan that the links are fastened between freight cars. Move the engine and the first car forward, and the whole train follows—if there is steam enough. It is much the same with the intercostal muscles. Move the first pair of ribs upward and the rest follow. Thus each rib is used to raise the one below it, and the whole rib framework goes up or down at the same time.

The external intercostals are the outer muscles of this class. There are eleven of these external inter-

costals on each side of the chest. The first intercostal
is between the first and second ribs, the second external
intercostal between the second and third ribs, and so
on down the bony trellis of the chest. Each of these
muscles has its origin, or starting point, at the lower
edge of the rib from which it proceeds, and its insertion,
or finishing point, at the upper edge of the rib next
below.

The internal intercostal muscles are the same in
number. Their origin is at the sternum, or breast
bone, and from the ridge on the inner surface of each
rib. The insertion of the internal intercostals is always
on the upper border of the rib below. The direction of
these internal intercostals is obliquely from the breast
bone toward the sides of the body—exactly opposite
to the direction taken by the external intercostals.

The serratus magnus muscle is a thin, irregular,
four-sided sheet of muscle. It lies close to the ribs.
It has its origin in nine thin slips of muscles that arise
from the eight upper ribs, there being two of these
slips attached to the second rib. This muscle extends
across to the shoulder, and the insertion is at the
scapula, or shoulder blade. This muscle, found on
either side of the chest, is used to assist in raising the
ribs.

Both the intercostals and the serratus magnus are
strengthened by deep breathing, and are greatly helped,
also, by any form of exercise that benefits the pectoral
muscles.

In the way of direct exercise it is to the pectorals
that the attention of the gymnast must be directed.
"Pectoral" may be translated as "chest." These
pectoral muscles are of two kinds, the major and the
minor.

The major pectoral muscle is a broad, thick muscle, triangular in shape. It covers the upper and fore part of the chest. It has its origin on the front of that half of the collar bone which is nearer the breast bone; and it also arises from the front side of the breast bone as far down as the point where the cartilage attaches to the sixth or the seventh rib. This muscle is also attached, by way of origin, to the cartilages of all of the upper seven ribs; although frequently it is not attached to the cartilages of either the first or the seventh rib, and sometimes to the cartilages of neither. The different portions of this muscle converge gradually, giving to it a fanlike shape. All portions of the muscle terminate, finally, in a tendon about two inches wide that is attached to the outer ridge of the humerus, the bone of the upper arm, and just at the base of the shoulder. The play of this tendon, and of the portion of the muscle near it, may be felt by moving the shoulder strongly backward and forward. In the same way, the movement of this muscle across the chest may be felt by the curious examiner.

The purpose of the major pectoral muscle is to draw the arm forward and across the chest. Thus, in general, exercises that force this motion will benefit the muscle. On a cold day it is a familiar sight to see a driver slapping his arms across his chest in an effort to warm himself by increasing circulation of the blood. This familiar movement is the most typical example of Nature's definite use of the muscle. In throwing your arms about a person, you exercise the same muscle. In climbing a rope or a ladder the pectoralis major is one of the muscles that is much employed; as it is in the raising or lowering of a flag or a sail. The same muscle must be used on one side of the body in sighting a gun. Driving generally gives this muscle some employment. So does rowing. An habitual oarsman is certain to have his major pectorals well developed, especially if he be careful to give both arms plenty of the exercise. By way of an industrial employment mowing with a scythe is an ideal form of exercise, or would be if farmers could but learn to use the scythe impartially on either side of the body, instead of, as is usually the case, only on the right. By way of sport, wrestling gives splendid exercise for this muscle.

In order to examine this muscle, and its gradual development, place the palm of the hand on the back of the neck with the point of the elbow extending sideways and about on a level with the shoulder. Then, by fairly rapid movements, force the elbow alternately far back and far forward. With the hand of the other arm, feel for the size and the motion of the major pectoral that is being exercised. Test the amount of development from time to time, by noting improvement in the size and hardness of this muscle.

There is another and excellent and simple way of testing the increasing strength of this muscle. If you have, or can obtain a pulley and rope, get an assortment of weights—flat-irons are about as handy as anything. Now, stand with, say, your left side toward the rope. Have a certain number of flat-irons attached to the weight-end of the rope. Now, hoisting the weights clear of the floor, and holding in your left hand the other end of the rope with your arm stretched out horizontally sideways toward the pulley, begin to move your hand inward until it touches your breast bone. Then straighten the arm out horizontally sideways again, and repeat this movement of straightening the arm and then touching the hand to the breast bone, several times. If you find that you can handle the amount of weight that is attached to the other end of the rope with a great deal of ease while doing this exercise, increase the amount of weight, bit by bit, until you find the amount that causes fatigue in doing the exercise. When you have reached what you find to be the limit of weight for performing this exercise without strain, note the amount of weight involved. A fortnight later, make the test again, noting with care how much more we ght you are able to handle than you did at the former test. Keep up these tests with fair frequency until you find, at last, that no amount of exercise will enable you to handle more than a certain weight. Then you will know that you have reached the probable limit of development of the left major pectoral.

Test the right major pectoral in the same way, by standing with the right side toward the pulley arrangement and holding the rope in the right hand. Note with care whether you are becoming stronger in the pectoral muscle of one side than in the same muscle on the other side. If so, exercise the weaker pectoral more than the stronger one, and keep this up until the respective strengths of the two pectorals are equal. It is a great mistake to develop one side of the body more than the other.

And now we come to a brief consideration of the minor pectoral. This is a thin muscle, flat and triangular in shape. It has its origin in the third, fourth and fifth ribs, near their cartilages. These portions of the muscle converge into a thin, flat tendon that is inserted at the inner border of the upper surface of the coracoid process. This coracoid process is a bony projection, shaped much like a crow's beak, at the front side of the shoulder blade. It helps to form the socket into which the upper end of the the upper arm bone, or humerus, fits.

The minor pectoral lies beneath the major pectoral, and hence its workings cannot be easily followed by the amateur investigator. The purpose of the minor pectoral is to depress the point of the shoulder; hence the best test of the gradually increasing strength of this muscle will be found by standing with the back to the pulley arrangement already described. Take the other end of the rope in one hand, raising that hand over the head. Step forward enough to lift the weights clear of the floor. Now, without bending the trunk, bring the engaged hand down across the chest until it touches the front upper leg on the other side of the body. Then return the hand over the head on its own side of the body. Repeat this several times. At every test, use all of the weight that you can without straining. As you are gradually able to use more and more weight at the other end of the rope, you will know that the strength of the minor pectoral is increasing.

CHAPTER VI.

Exercises for Developing the Muscles of the Chest.

The photographs, numbers 3, 4, 5 and 6, illustrate the best kinds of exercise for developing the muscles of the chest to the utmost. Study them well and practice them with a full remembrance of what I said of the uses of these muscles, and you will realize the application and value of the exercises.

Take, for instance, exercise number three, as shown in photographs numbers 3 and 4. In this, after an intelligent trial, you will realize that the hooking of the fingers and the ensuing tug is bound to benefit the major pectoral muscles, for here you are forcing each arm to do the work of crossing the chest. In raising the arms forward you are also exercising the major pectorals. At the same time, in starting, the shoulder points are naturally a trifle depressed. This gradual change from a position of shoulder points depressed to one with the points well backward, gives its true work, in an emphatic form, to the minor pectorals.

At the conclusion of the movement both sets of pectorals have been exercised in a thorough manner— *if!* And on this "if" hangs the secret of success with this exercise. There must be as much strength as possible used in the work. You can do this work lightly and with corresponding lack of benefit. So put vim, strength and *attention* into the work. Remember

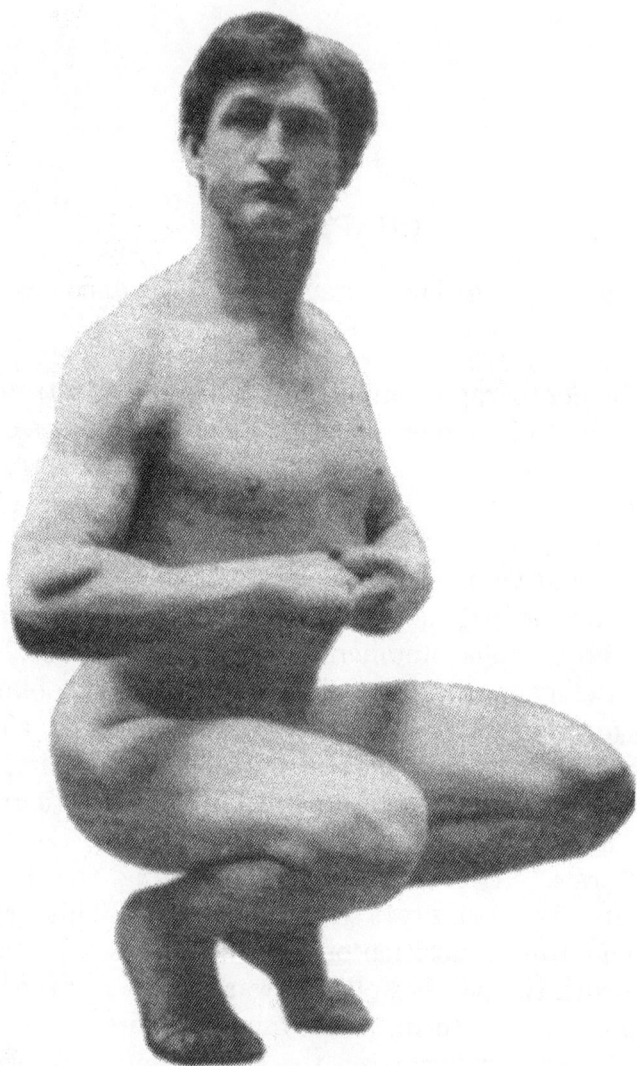

Photograph No. 3.

Exercise No. 3. Form one finger of each hand like a hook; then locking them together and balancing the body on the toes, as shown in the photo, slowly raise the arms forward and upward, all the time pulling vigorously outward and attempting to pull the fingers apart. (See next photo.)

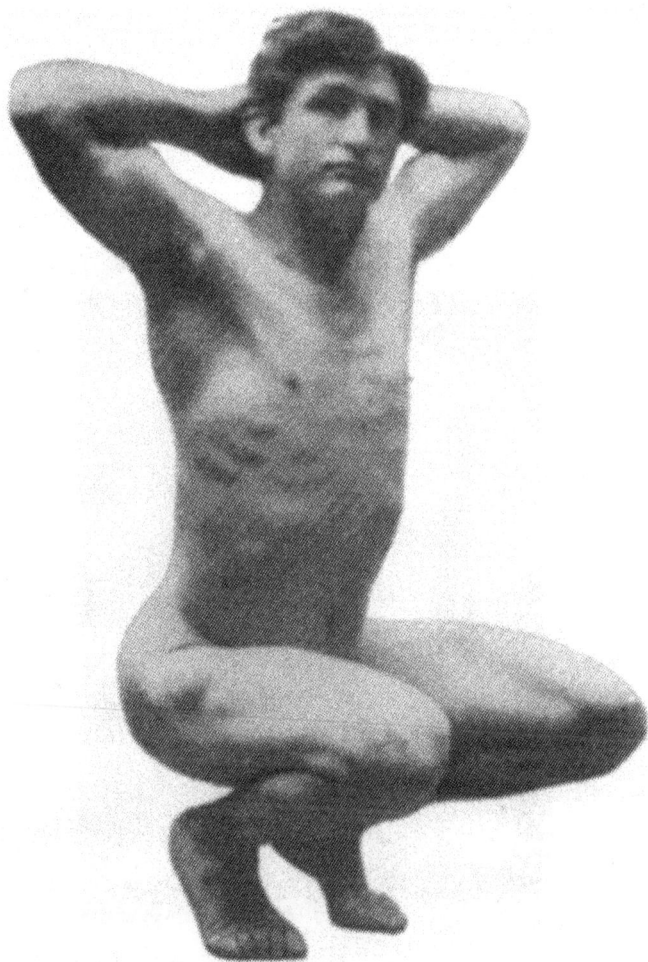

Photograph No. 4.

Continue to slowly draw the arms upward until they are
far back of the head, as shown in the above photo. Be sure to
make vigorous effort to pull the fingers apart while bringing the
arms upward. Use each of the fingers of both hands in this
manner. This is a very good all-round exerciser for strengthening the fingers, arms, chest and legs. As a variation, if desired,
you can raise up and go down by straightening the knees. If
you have difficulty in maintaining your balance while taking
this exercise, when first attempting it, you can lean against a
chair or table. This exercise is also especially good for rounding
the knees and for making the legs shapely.

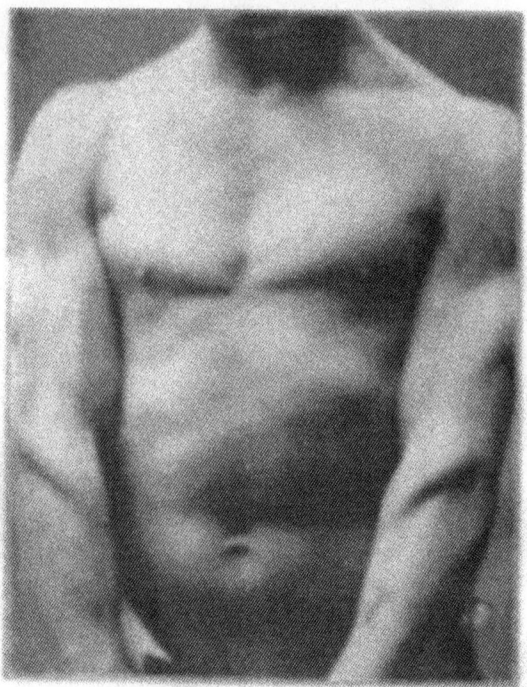

Photograph No. 5.

Exercise No. 4. Bring the shoulders downward and as far forward as you can. Now slowly bring them backward and upward. (See next photo.)

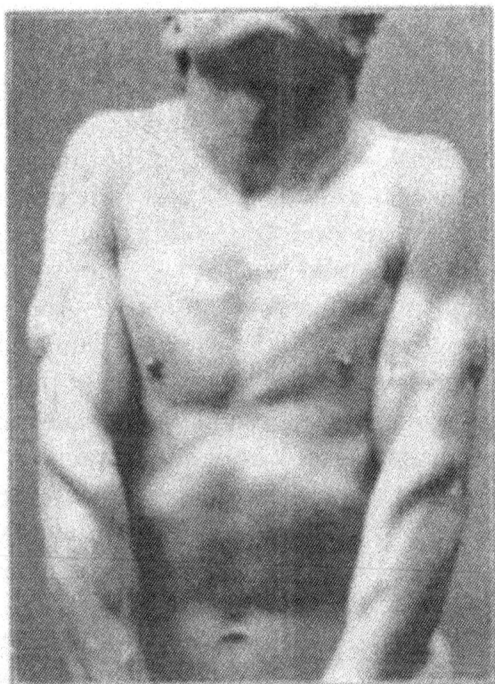

Photograph No. 6.

To position shown above, throwing the head as far back as you can at the same time. This exercise is especially beneficial in straightening round shoulders, and it should be repeated until tired, two or three times a day, if bothered with a defect of this nature. The exercise can be made still more difficult if you will, after having brought the shoulders up and back as far as you can, make two or three attempts to bring them still farther back and down as far as you can.

that every time you perform the movement weakly or slightingly, you have been careless enough to waste so much of the time that you have to devote to your muscular development.

Yet, take care that you do not make the mistake that some of my readers are sure to make. Do not imagine that these chest exercises are of but comparatively little importance. Do not try these only now and then, giving most of your time to making your biceps larger. Fine biceps are splendid but they are not by any means the key to all muscular development. And remember that the practical strength of your arms will fall far below your proper standard if you do not pay attention to the vigorous development of your chest muscles.

Now, let us take a look at exercise number four, as it is shown in photographs numbers 5 and 6. Study the photographs well, and get a good mental grasp of the text. When you have done this, try the exercise—not in a lackadaisical way, but with strength and purpose. Put all of your normal power into the work. Then, when you have noted the effect, think over what I have written in the preceding chapter concerning the main purpose of the minor pectoral muscle.

Do you now comprehend the full meaning of this exercise? By starting with the shoulders well downward and forward, and by slowly forcing them backward and upward against the strong resistance of other muscles, you strengthen the minor pectorals for the natural muscular work that they have to do in depressing the points of the shoulders. And, after faithful practice of this exercise for some time, say every day for two or three weeks, you will be astonished at the increase of your strength in these little-heard-of but very important muscles.

No matter how strong you become, these exercises for the chest muscles should be continued zealously and faithfully.

It is important to remember that a measure of interest and pleasure in the performance of your exercises will result in a vastly more marked benefit than their execution in an indifferent or perfunctory manner.   Herein lies the explanation of the failure of the manual laborer, whose muscles obey the mandates of his mind only under protest, to secure the development of the athlete, from the standpoint of either symmetry or endurance.   You will gain more strength from a few energet c, concentrated efforts than from a thousand listless, sluggish movements.   Furthermore, you will be able to enjoy every exercise if you enter into it vigorously.   And if you can thus make your exercises appeal to you in the form of play, so much the better.

CHAPTER VII.

Anatomical Structure of the Shoulders.

Certainly the shoulder is one of the dominating parts of the body. We say that a man has "broad shoulders," and this instantly calls up the picture of a massive frame, great strength and enviable endurance. We say of one that he has "put his shoulder to the wheel"— and this conveys the impression that the wheel will have to move. The shoulders have ever been the burden bearers. Men even elevate the popular hero on to their shoulders. In industry, a man is "up to his shoulders" in work. But we have yet to find a phrase in which the shoulders are associated with indolence.

At first thought, the anatomical structure of the shoulder is strange. The basis of the shoulder is the scapula, or shoulder blade. This is a flat, triangular bone with its greatest length pointing downward. In front, the bone terminates in a beak-shaped projection that is known as the coracoid process. At the back of the scapula is a long, narrow spine that ends in a projection of bone called the acromion process. It is in the cavity or socket formed by the coracoid and acromion processes that the round, ball-like head of the humerus, or bone of the upper arm fits and moves. This cavity between the two processes is known as the glenoid cavity.

Now, consider how this highly important shoulder blade is held in place. It is attached to the clavicle or collar bone, that thin little bone that runs across the front of the chest to the sternum or breast bone. Outside of this, the attachment of the shoulder blade to the trunk is chiefly by means of muscles. It will be understood, then, that when these muscles are strong and active, a great variety of movements of the shoulders are possible, and much power lies behind these movements.

In all, seventeen different muscles are attached, in a greater or less degree, to the shoulder blade. Among these are some of the most powerful muscles in the body. I am not going to weary you with the names and descriptions of all the seventeen, but it will be worth while to note some of the more important muscles that depend largely upon the shoulder for their effectiveness.

First of all, there is the deltoid muscle, a true shoulder muscle of which I shall say more a little further on. The serratus magnus, which I described in Chapter V., is another of the muscles that are attached to the scapula. The rhomboids, minor and major, those powerful and effective muscles of the back, have much of their play across the shoulder blade, and are attached to it. The triceps and biceps, those most powerful and useful of the muscles of the upper arm, are secured to the shoulder blade, and so is the minor pectoral muscle, of which I spoke in Chapter V. In fact, there are few applied movements of the trunk in which the shoulders do not play a leading part.

Even as a guard against injury from accident, it is important to have shoulders that show the best possible development. We do not often hear of cases of the shoulder-blade being fractured, but fractures of the rather fragile collar bone are common enough. A severe fall upon the shoulder very often results in a broken collar bone.   Were the shoulder well developed, the collar bone would have a much better chance of safety.

Drooping shoulders show lack of uniform development at this point.   True, a round-shouldered man may have very strong muscles; but if all of the muscles of the shoulder and those attached to the shoulder blade were properly developed, the man's carriage would be as erect and graceful as Nature intended it to be.

It is an ample indication of the far-reaching effects of proper shoulder development to state that usually even a few fibres of the latissimus dorsi, that powerful muscle of the lower back, are found to be attached to one of the angles of the scapula.

Can you find, then, any better single point of the body at which the muscular structure should be of the toughest and most durable?   For even the biceps and the triceps, those powerful striking and lifting muscles of the arm, must depend on the shoulders for much of their strength.

It is in the deltoid muscle that we find the true shoulder muscle, that which covers and serves the shoulder alone.   This muscle can be felt easily on the outside of the shoulder.   The deltoid's work is to move the arm out at the side and upward.   Hence any motion of the arm that is accomplished with sufficient vigor and resistance belongs to the exercises that are to be used in the strengthening of the deltoid muscle.

The deltoid is a large muscle, as it must be to cover the shoulder.   It is thick and triangular and is so moulded over the shoulder that, in its best development, it gives the roundness and the beauty of contour that lovers of the perfect human figure demand.

The origin of this deltoid muscle is three-fold. It arises from the front border and upper surface of the outer third of the collar bone—that is, of the third of the collar bone that is nearer the shoulder blade; it arises also from the outer margin and upper sur face of the acromion process; and furthermore from the rear border of the spine that runs along the back of the scapula. The fibres of the muscle converge until they unite in a tough, thick tendon that is inserted in a rough triangular ridge of bone at the middle of the outer side of the shaft of the humerus or bone of the upper arm. By studying the origin, position and insertion of this muscle you will understand how, in a well-developed state, it is fitted to do its work to wonderful advantage.

The simplest test for the strength of the deltoid muscle, and for watching the gradual increase in its strength, is to be found by grasping a light weight in the hand. Stand with the hand at the side of the leg. Now, raise the arm slowly and steadily outward at the side, keeping the arm straight all the while, and continue this raising sideways until the hand is up over the head. If you find that the work with the weight chosen is altogether too easily done, take a somewhat heavier weight and repeat the test. It will not take you long to discover just how much weight your deltoid muscle is capable of lifting. In comparative tests thereafter, note the increase in weight that you are able to lift from time to time, and it is of decided advantage to keep a record of such improvement.

Be careful to exercise the deltoids of each shoulder impartially, unless the tests show that one deltoid is considerably stronger than the other. In that case, give the weaker deltoid more exercise than its fellow until the inequality is overcome.

CHAPTER VIII.

Exercises for Developing the Muscles of the Shoulders.

For the important work of developing the shoulders there are four exercises that should be undertaken with a great deal of regularity. These exercises are illustrated by eight photographs, and the meaning of each step in this exercise work will be plain.

Do not go at these exercises laggingly. Like everything else that is worth doing at all, these exercises are worth doing well. Make every movement firmly and strongly, and see that the other and antagonistic muscles are made to resist the efforts of the muscles that you are exercising.

Make frequent tests of the improvement in strength in your shoulders. Do not be satisfied with a stationary condition of strength. If you do not gradually grow a great deal stronger in the shoulders there is sure to be some mistake in the way that you are doing the exercises. Either you are not following directions closely, or you are not employing enough strength and vim in the work, or you are taking up particular exercises with too little frequency. Find out the weak spot in your work and eradicate it.

Exercise number five, as shown in photographs numbers 7 and 8, will give you an excellent idea of the resistant work. It gives you also an opportunity to understand exactly what I mean by "strong resistant work." First of all, perform the exercise with very ordinary resistance on the part of the left hand and arm. Next move the right arm back against the very strongest resistance of which your left hand and arm is capable.

It is this strong resistance that constitutes the very essence of the work. Unless the resistance is made very hard and firm you are wasting most of the time that you employ on the work!

The same remarks hold true of exercise number six, which is illustrated by the photographs numbers 9 and 10. Here there is scope for exercise so severe that at first you can make it lame your back. Of course, I do not mean that any student of physical training should strain his muscles too severely, but the danger will all lie in the other direction—that of too light work. Do not lame your back and arms badly; but at the outset do not be surprised if you do make the muscles a trifle sore. All athletic work, when first undertaken, has this effect. The lameness gradually disappears through the strengthening of the muscles that were formerly weak.

Exercise number seven, which is fully explained by photographs numbers 11 and 12, offers some work that brings the deltoids most excellently and strongly into play. Do not be afraid of laming your deltoids. You will have to do the work severely, or you will not secure the development that you want for this part of the body. Remember that the deltoids have a way of doing their work in a lazy and perfunctory manner if they are not watched. Very few men have well-developed deltoids. This particular exercise, if it is faithfully used, will make you strong where most men are weak.

Exercise number eight, illustrated by photographs numbers 13 and 14, will continue the good work for the indolent deltoids. It will bring out a firmer, sounder, stronger pad of muscle right at the central portion of the slope in the shoulders.

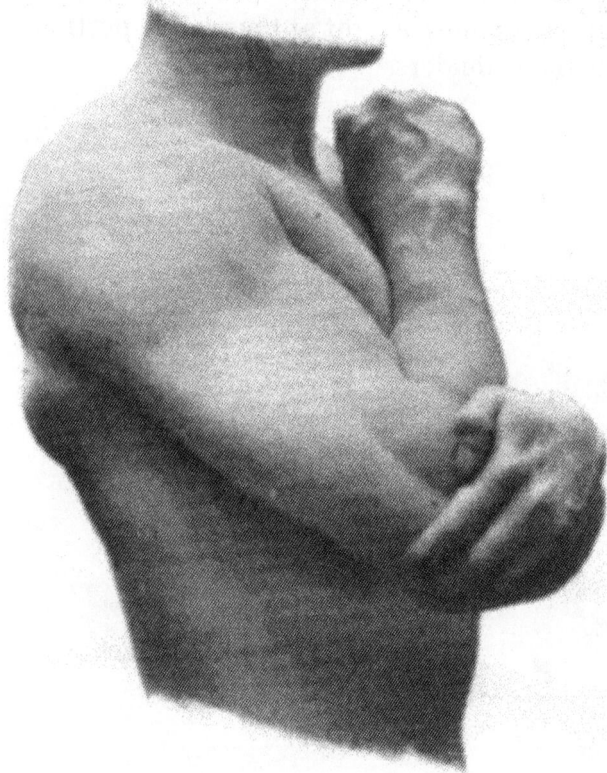

Photograph No. 7.

Exercise No. 5. Grasp the right elbow with the left hand, as shown in photo. Now bring the right arm downward and backward (See next photo).

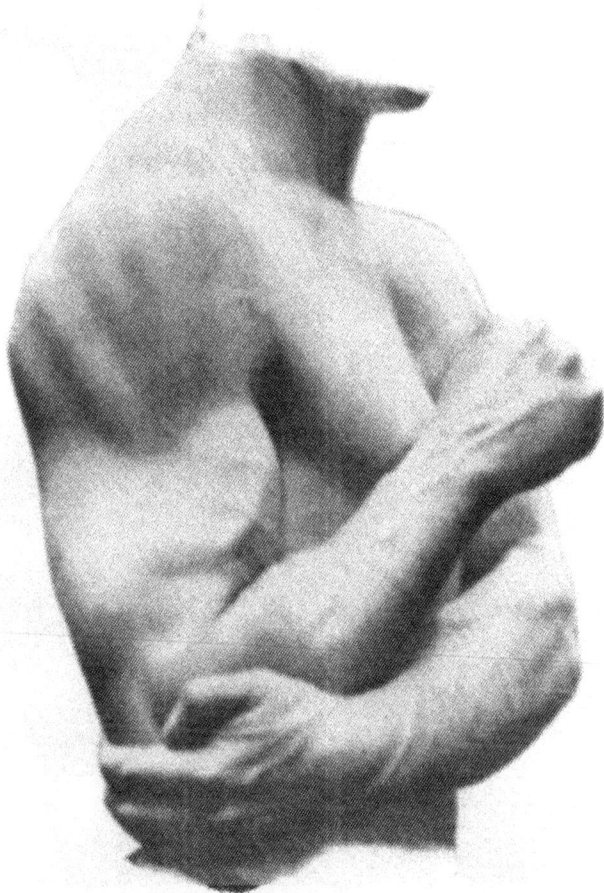

Photograph No. 8.

To position shown in this photo. While the right arm goes downward and backward, resist vigorously the movements with the left arm, making it require considerable effort to bring the arm back to the position shown. Take similar exercise with the left arm, reversing the position until the muscles are thoroughly tired. This exercise is for strengthening and developing the muscles in the back part of the shoulder.

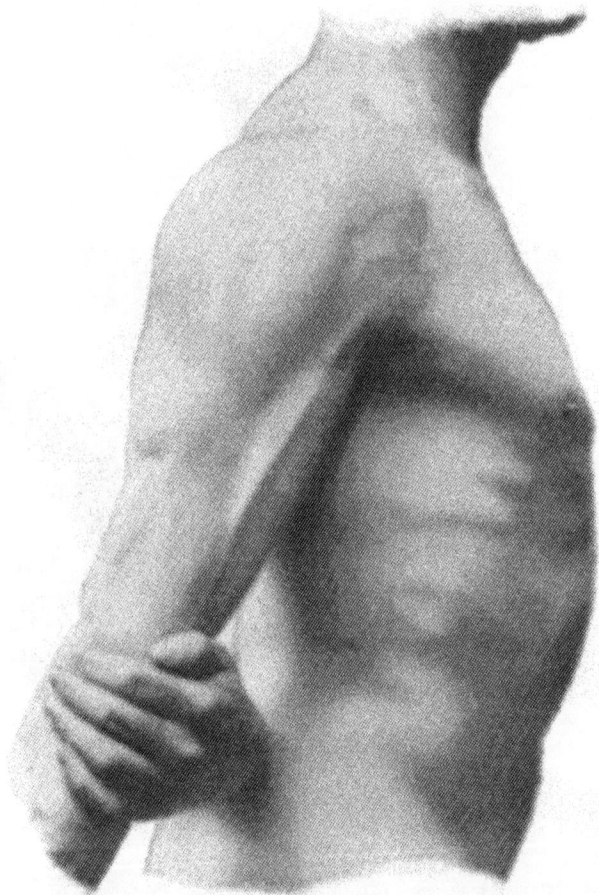

Photograph No. 9.

Exercise No. 6. Grasp the right arm with the left hand behind the back, as shown in the illustration. Now, strongly resisting the movement with the left arm, bring the right arm forward as far as you can (See next photo).

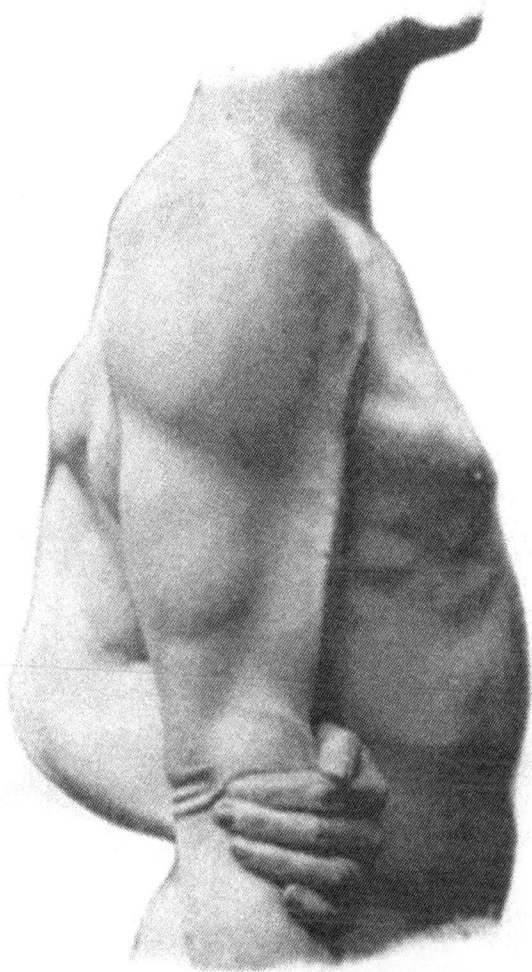

Photograph No. 10.

To position shown in this photograph. Continue the exercises until the muscles are thoroughly tired, being sure to resist the movements vigorously each time. Take same exercises with both arms, reversing the position. This movement strengthens and develops the muscles in the front part of the shoulder.

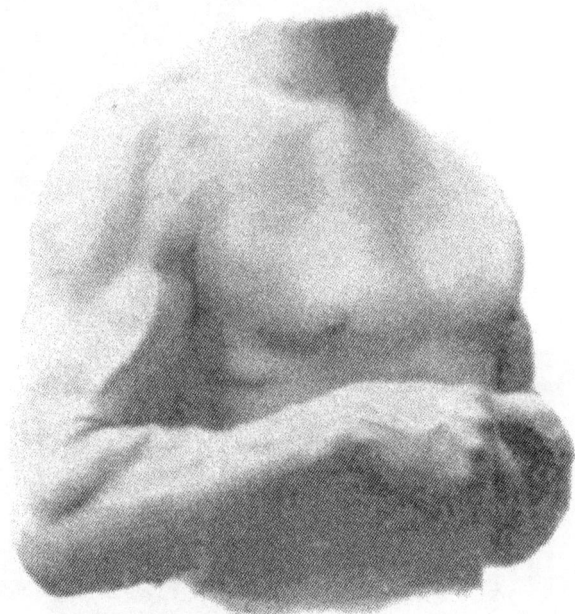

Photograph No. 11.

Exercise No. 7. Grasp the hands as shown in the photograph. Now bring the right arm outward and upward at the side (See next photo).

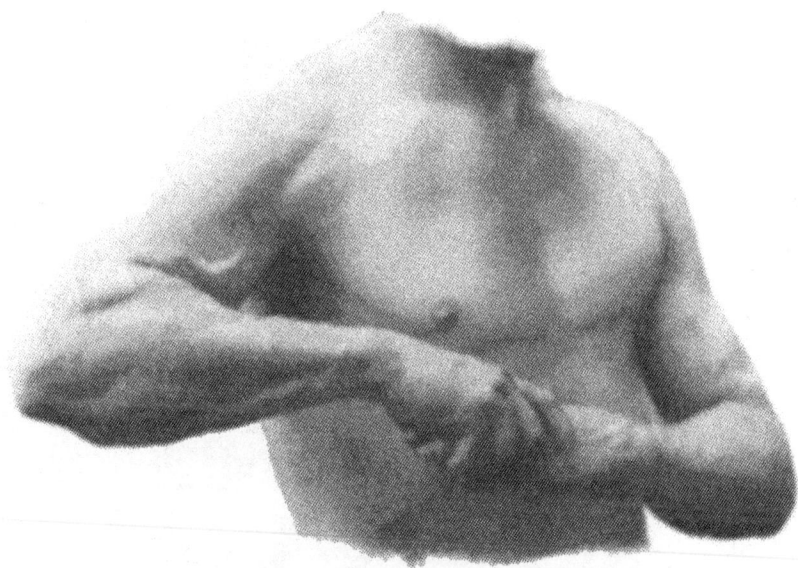

Photograph No. 12.

To position shown in this photograph. Strongly resist
the movement of the right arm with the left, then reverse the
movement, bringing the left arm out at the side and resisting
with the right arm. Continue this exercise until the muscles
on the sides of each shoulder are thoroughly tired; and if you
are taking the exercise properly this will not require very many
movements. This movement is for strengthening and develor·
ing the muscles on the outer part of the shoulder.

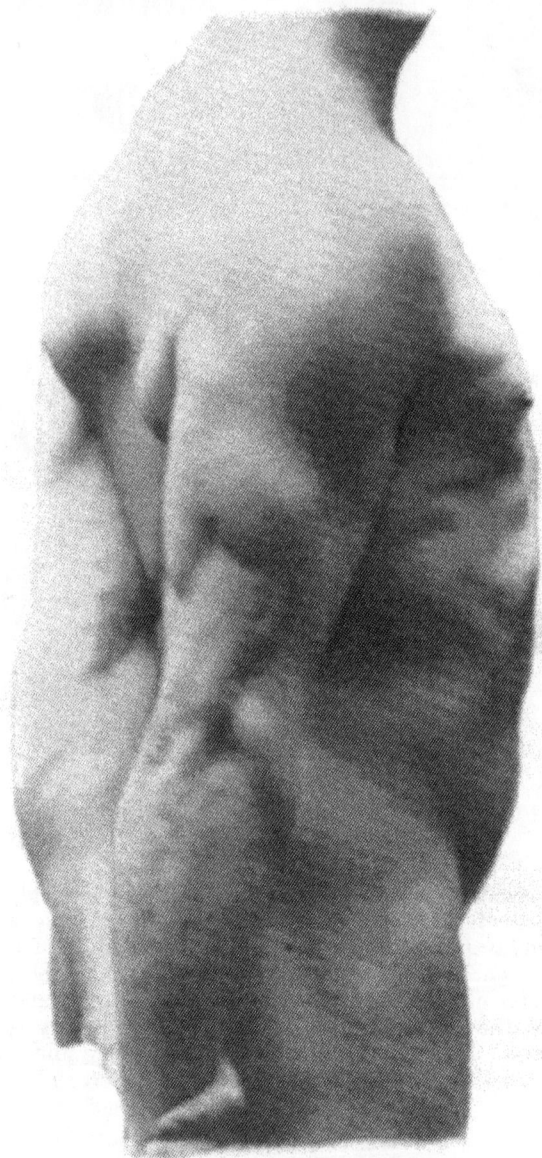

Photograph No. 13.

Exercise No. 8. Grasp the right wrist with the left hand as shown in photograph. Now, while pulling downward vigorously with the left arm, raise the right shoulder as high as you can. (See next photo.)

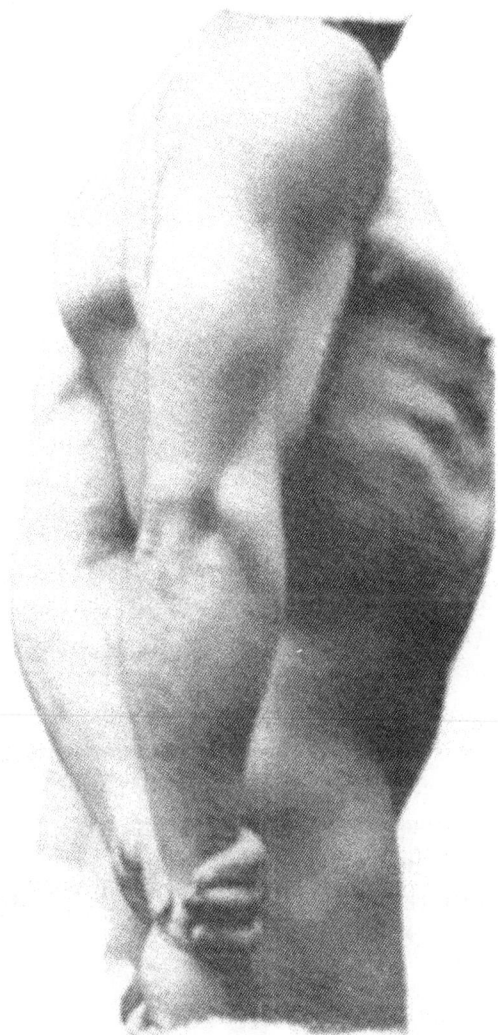

Photograph No. 14.

As shown in the above photograph, the shoulders should be raised each time as high as you can make them go. Continue the exercise until the muscles are tired; then reverse the position and take same exercise with the right hand grasping the left wrist. This exercise is especially advantageous in developing the muscles in the central portion of the slope of shoulders.

CHAPTER IX.

ANATOMICAL STRUCTURE OF THE UPPER ARM.

In the upper arm there are two muscles of great importance. Of one of these everyone who has ever tried to increase his muscular powers knows the nature. This is the biceps muscle. There is another, the triceps, which is equally important, and which does work exactly the opposite to that performed by biceps.

Before describing any of the muscles of the upper arm, however, I shall devote a little space to remark on its general anatomical structure. As probably every one of my readers knows, there is but one bone in the upper arm. This is the humerus, and it corresponds very closely to the thigh bone of the upper leg. The humerus shaft extends from the elbow to the shoulder blade. At the shoulder is the rounded head of the humerus, which, as explained in Chapter VII, fits nicely into the glenoid cavity, or socket between the acromion and coracoid processes of the scapula or shoulder blade. This fitting-in of the head of the humerus to the glenoid cavity supplies a ball and socket mechanism that is at the same time simple and wonderful. A fluid is supplied to the cavity that makes it possible for the head of the humerus to move about without creating friction. The humerus is held in place by the attachments of various muscles.

The biceps muscle is so-called because it is two-headed; that is, it has its origin at two separate points, and really begins as two separate muscles, which combine further on to form one general muscle.   This is the flexor muscle of the arm, or the muscle that causes the arm to "flex."   By "flexing" we mean the bending of the fore-arm over upon the upper arm.   It is the muscle employed in lifting anything, or in hauling, tugging, but not in striking a straight-arm blow.

The shorter head of the biceps arises in a thick, flat tendon that proceeds from the point of the coracoid process, while the longer head rises from the upper margin of the glenoid cavity.   This latter tendon arches over the head of the humerus.   Each tendon develops into a long "belly" of muscle, and these bellies can easily be separated until they reach a point within about three inches of the elbow joint.   Here they become firmly combined as one muscle.   Then too, the muscle is tightly twisted.   The insertion is through a flat tendon that is attached to a prominence on the radius, or smaller bone of the lower arm.   It will be understood, therefore, how perfectly the biceps is placed for its work of flexing the arm.

Occasionally—and according to some authorities as often as once in every eight or ten cases—there is found to be a third head to the biceps, and this head may consist of either one or two slips of tendon.

From the fact that it has three heads, or points of origin, the triceps receives its name.   This is the extensor muscle of the upper arm, and its work, in contrast with the function of the biceps, is to extend the arm—that is, to straighten it out again after the biceps has flexed it.   Thus it will be seen that the biceps plays really no part in delivering a straight-arm blow, this task falling upon the triceps.   But as the biceps and triceps must be trained in symmetry, and whatever exercises one muscle is sure to benefit the other muscle, it will be understood' that the training of biceps and triceps must go on simultaneously, and with, in nearly all kinds of exercise, equal benefit.   In fact, it would be an anomaly for a man to possess splendidly developed biceps and an infinitely weaker triceps.

These three heads of the triceps are known as the middle, scapular or long head; the external or long humeral; and the internal, or short humeral.   The scapular head has its origin in a flat tendon proceeding from a triangular indentation on the scapula and just below the glenoid cavity.   The external or long humeral head is a tendon that has its starting point mainly from the outside border of the humerus, while the internal head has its starting point on the rear surface of the shaft of the humerus.

While the triceps covers the entire length of the rear surface of the humerus, the muscle begins to take on a tendinous form—that is, begins to change from what we commonly consider as muscular tissue into the harder substance of the tendon—at about the middle of the back part of the muscle.   At this beginning of the tendon there are two portions, one close to the surface and the other much more deeply imbedded in the muscle.   They join together just above the elbow, and the insertion of this triceps tendon is mainly in the back portion of the upper surface of the olecranon process— the eminence of bone at the upper and back part of the ulna or principal bone of the forearm.   This process is what is commonly called the point of the elbow, and we can easily feel its contour when we bend the arm. We can also, by alternately flexing and extending the arm, feel the workings of the tendon at the point of its insertion in the olecranon process. From this description it will be easy to understand how the triceps muscle is admirably situated for its task of extending the arm.

Closely connected with the heads of the biceps is the subscapularis muscle, which is situated at the head of the arm in the region where the biceps originates. The insertion is in the humerus on the biceps side of the shaft. This subscapularis muscle is a large and triangular shaped affair, and plays an important part in raising the arm.

Then we have to consider the coraco-brachialis muscle, which arises mainly from the coracoid process. This is a small muscle, yet an important one. It is situated at the upper and inner part of the arm, and its workings may be very plainly defined through the flesh. Its insertion is by means of a flat tendon into an impression on the inner surface of the humerus at about the middle of the upper arm.

Then there is a muscle to which I wish to call the particular attention of my readers, since its existence in a firm, well-developed state is one of the sure indications of a thoroughly muscular arm. This is the brachialis anticus. It covers the elbow joint and the lower half of the front side of the humerus. In bending the arm and at the same time bringing the fist in front of the chest, this muscle if well built, stands out prominently on the upper side of the elbow. It should be prominent, well knotted and "hard as a rock." It has its origin from the lower half of the outer and inner surfaces of the shaft of the humerus, just above the insertion of the deltoid muscle. This origin extends to within about an inch of the elbow joint. The insertion of this muscle is by a thick tendon in the head of the ulna, or larger bone of the forearm.

All of the muscles that I have described in the foregoing will be prominently outlined in the true athletic arm. And if these muscles be well developed the improvement of the lesser muscles is bound to follow while other lesser muscles which have not been mentioned, may be left to take care of themselves, sharing as they must, in the benefits received by the more important muscles.

About the easiest test for the strength of the biceps is to note how heavy a weight—a dumbbell or anything else—can be held in the hand when the arm is flexed. Improvement in the strength of the biceps can be tested by noting the gradual increase in the amount of weight that can be held in the hand while completely flexing the arm.

About the simplest way of testing improvement in the triceps is found by practicing, from time to time, at the machine which registers the striking power of the arm. A very careful record should be kept of such improvement. If there is no improvement, or if it is so slight as to be discouraging, then the work for the triceps should be greatly increased.

Tests for improvement in the subscapularis, coracobrachialis and brachialis anticus muscles are not so simple. In fact, it is enough to remember that satisfactory improvement in the biceps and triceps indicates, in a general way, that the other three muscles are receiving the attention that they need.

It is to the biceps that the misinformed look first of all for indications of an athlete's probable capacity. While as a matter of fact, strong biceps are indeed absolutely necessary to the strong man, yet a word of caution in this respect is necessary. Most athletes give too much attention to the biceps, regarding it as the best "show" asset of the body. This is a mistake. The development of the whole muscular system should be uniform and symmetrical in the ideal strong man, and he is a wise athlete who does not devote the greater portion of his time to the acquiring of bulging biceps.

And do not lose sight of my hint that, in studying the gradual development of the upper arm, the condition and size of the brachialis anticus muscle must be watched carefully. Movements that bring the fists in across the chest when flexing the arm not only show up the brachialis anticus, but also afford exercise to this very valuable muscle.

With these remarks and cautions we will now proceed to the discussion of exercises that make for the muscular perfection of the upper arm.

CHAPTER X.

EXERCISES FOR DEVELOPING THE MUSCLES OF THE UPPER ARM.

Ten photographs are required to illustrate the five exercises that I shall offer for the making of the perfect upper arm. These exercises are all easy to learn, and if they are persisted in with vim, strength and snap, they will accomplish their end.

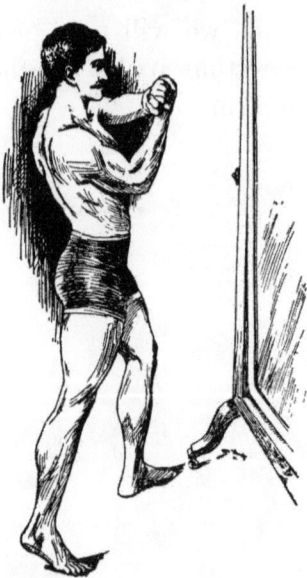

Your exercise can be made more interesting if you will stand before a mirror and watch the muscles as they are flexed and relaxed.

There is one hint that I wish to offer at this point. Acquire the habit of doing your exercising before a mirror. This not only enables you to watch your gradual development and to note just how it is brought about, but also makes the work pleasanter, and thereby relieves the tedium that is often encountered when exercise reaches the perfunctory stage

Exercise number nine, as shown in photographs 15 and 16, supplies when done just as directed, one of the of the most effective bits of

70

work that can possibly be. The biceps are brought forcefully into play, and it gives fine quality as well as size to this muscle. It will be noted in the photograph, too, that the brachialis anticus muscle stands well out. This is due to the fact that that muscle is much employed in this exercise, which constitutes another reason for the frequent employment of the latter.

Exercise number ten, illustrated by photographs 17 and 18, gives the triceps such strong work that at first, this and other muscles will be considerably lamed thereby. The coraco-brachialis and subscapularis, too, are strongly brought into play. If the biceps of the right arm be much better developed than that of the left, there will be a temptation to give the right arm added work in order to watch the play of the muscles. This is a mistake. If the right biceps be much better developed than the left, the proper course will be to give the left biceps more work until the inequality is overcome.

Exercise eleven, shown in photographs 19 and 20, gives simple but excellent employment for all of the muscles of the upper arm, except the triceps. Here too, the brachialis anticus muscle shares largely in the exertion of the biceps. The twisting movement gives both firmness and elasticity to the muscles that receive the most work. It is an all-around good exercise for the arm.

Exercise twelve does not give special work to any one muscle. It involves all of the muscles of the upper arm, and with the best possible results for a symmetrical, uniform development of the upper arm. It rapidly creates that might of arm of which hero-worshipping poets have ever been wont to sing. It brings out prominently the muscles that are used in work on the bars and flying rings.

Exercise thirteen, shown in photographs 23 and 24, will be of interest to all of my friends who have an enthusiastic respect for bulging biceps. It is, in fact, the exercise that develops the biceps most rapidly, but the brachialis anticus muscle over the elbow joint is not benefited to the same extent as in some of the other exercises.

Now, it is time to say a special word to my readers. You should learn to analyze all the movements through which you go in securing unusual muscular development. Do not perform the different forms of work simply because I advise the exercises. Learn to study for yourself just *what* muscles are benefited. Find out *just how* these muscles are affected. Then figure out the *why*.

If you are ever in doubt as to exactly what muscle is most affected by a certain exercise, there is one test that is quite reliable, and that is to carry some one exercise on some special occasion to such a limit that the after feeling will show you beyond a doubt just which muscle has been most directly concerned. Of course it is understood that in taking all exercises for building up increased muscular power, each movement should be continued until a tired feeling indicates that it has been carried far enough. And it is also understood that overwork and exhaustion is worse than no exercise at all. But it is possible to use some one special muscle to such an extent that the muscle itself will feel the effects of the work it has done, and yet without too great a constitutional effort, that is, without overtaxing the heart, lungs and other vital organs.

So that when you wish to experiment with this end

in view, simply continue the one movement, in which you are for the time interested, considerably longer than is your usual habit, carrying it to the point where the muscles being used actually ache. This aching will indicate very plainly just what you are trying to find out. Massage that part immediately afterward, however. If you are not satisfied with this you might repeat the experiment a few minutes later, and then again, with the result that you will have a stiff and lame muscle for a couple of days after to convince and remind you of your newly acquired knowledge.

Continue the analysis of your various athletic tasks until you understand the full nature of every exercise that you attempt. Then—and not until then—will you begin to be proficient in the development of the human body. Believe me, if you go at it in the right way, you can teach yourself more than I can teach you through the medium of printers ink.

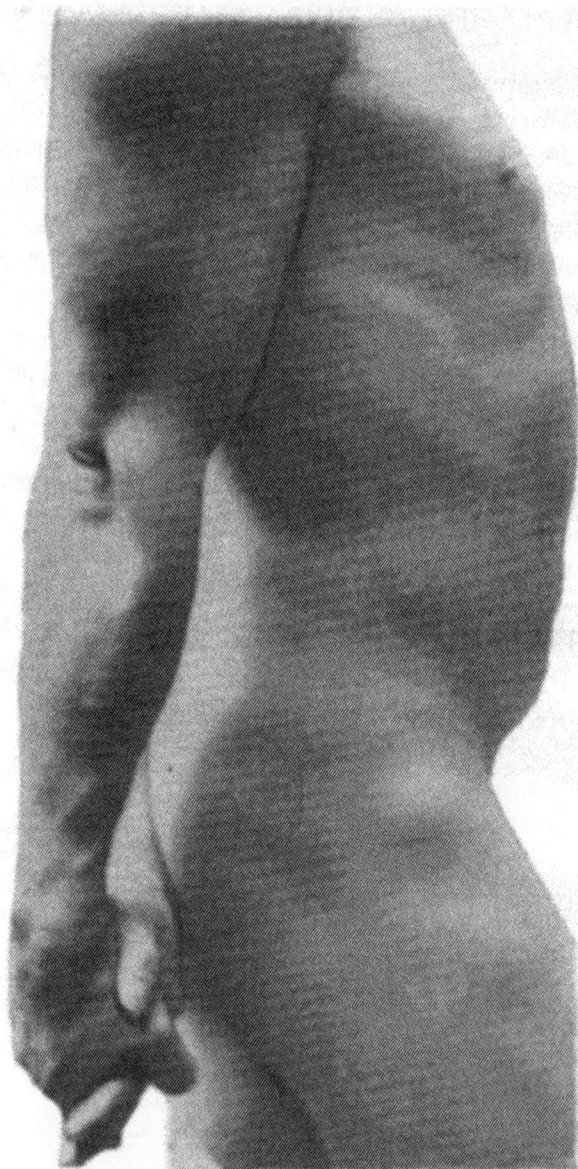

Photograph No. 15.

Exercise No. 9. Place the left hand in the right palm, as shown in the illustration. Now, resisting the movement slightly with the left hand, bring the (See next photo.)

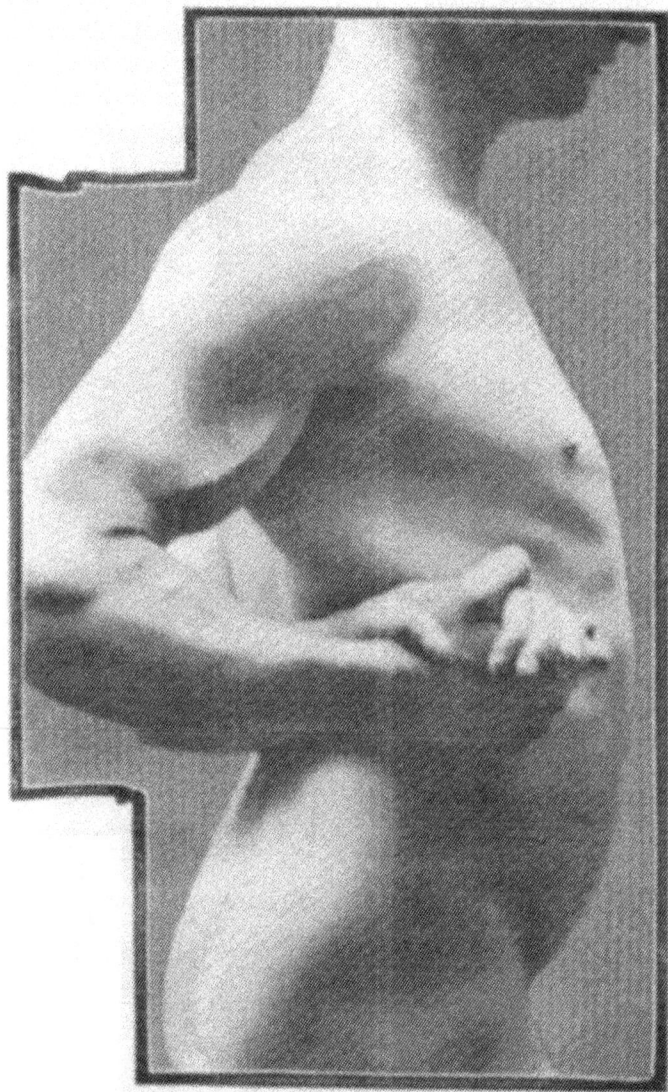

Photograph No. 16.

Right hand up and forward as far as you can, bending the arm, as shown in the above illustration. This is one of the most effective movements that can possibly be devised for bringing into thorough action the biceps—the largest muscle of the upper arm. This exercise can be varied slightly by placing the left hand on the back of the right hand, instead of in the palm. Take same exercise with position of arms and hands reversed. Continue the exercise with each arm until tired.

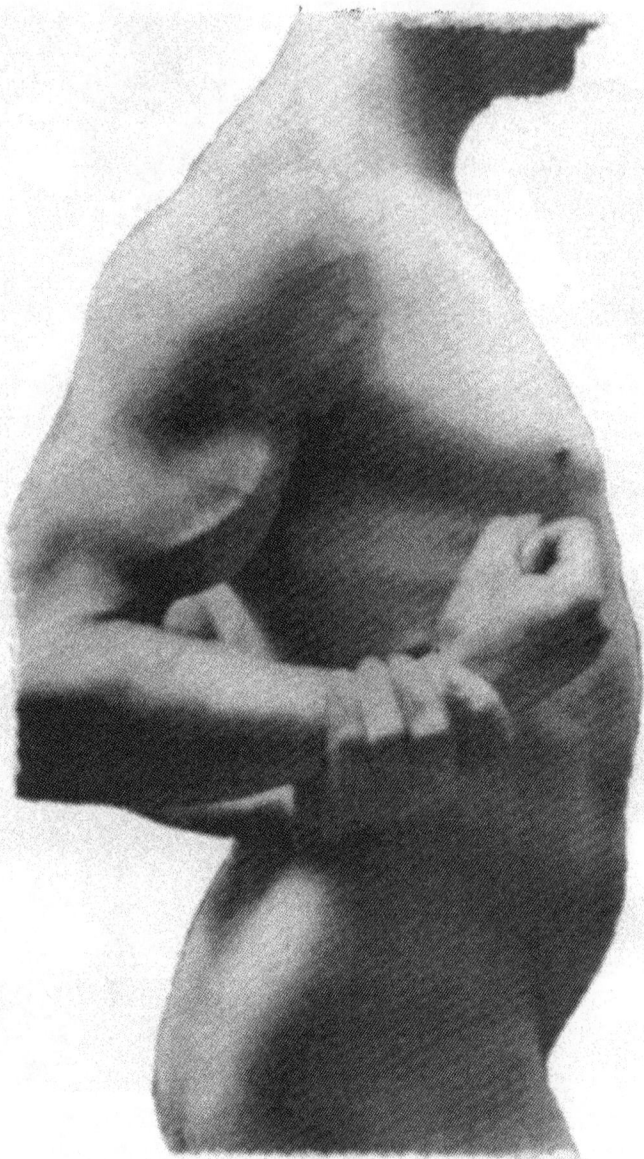

Photograph No. 17.

Exercise No. 10. Grasp the right wrist with the left hand, as shown in the illustration. Now, resisting the motion with the left hand, straighten the right arm, (See next photo.)

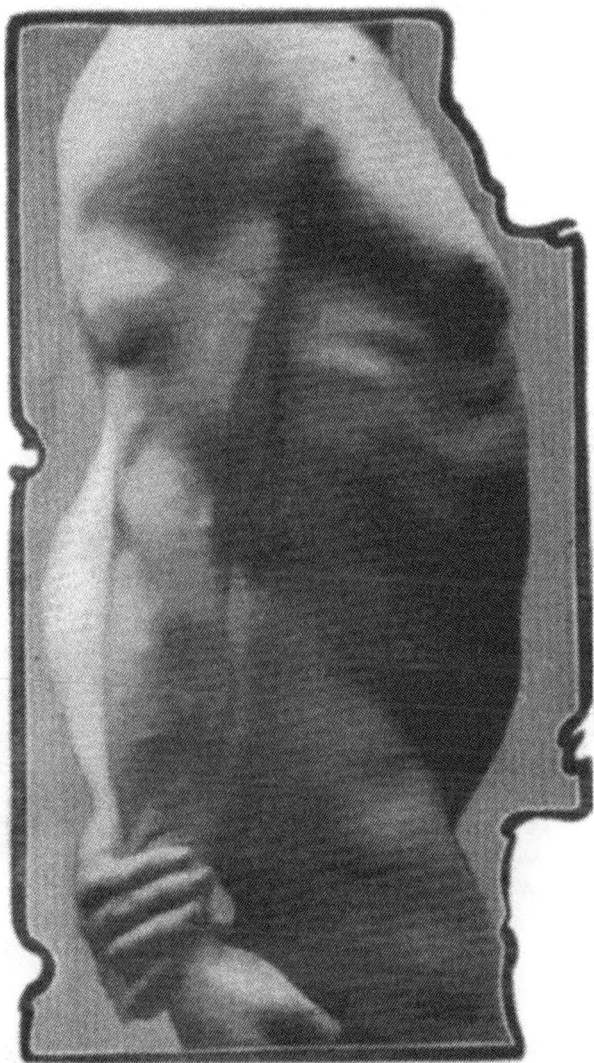

Photograph No. 18.

As shown in the above illustration. Be sure to bring the
right arm downward until entirely straight each time. This
exercise can be taken also with the palm turned downward.
Take same exercise, reversing employment of the arms and
hands. Continue the exercise with each arm until tired. For
the triceps, the large muscles that straighten arm.

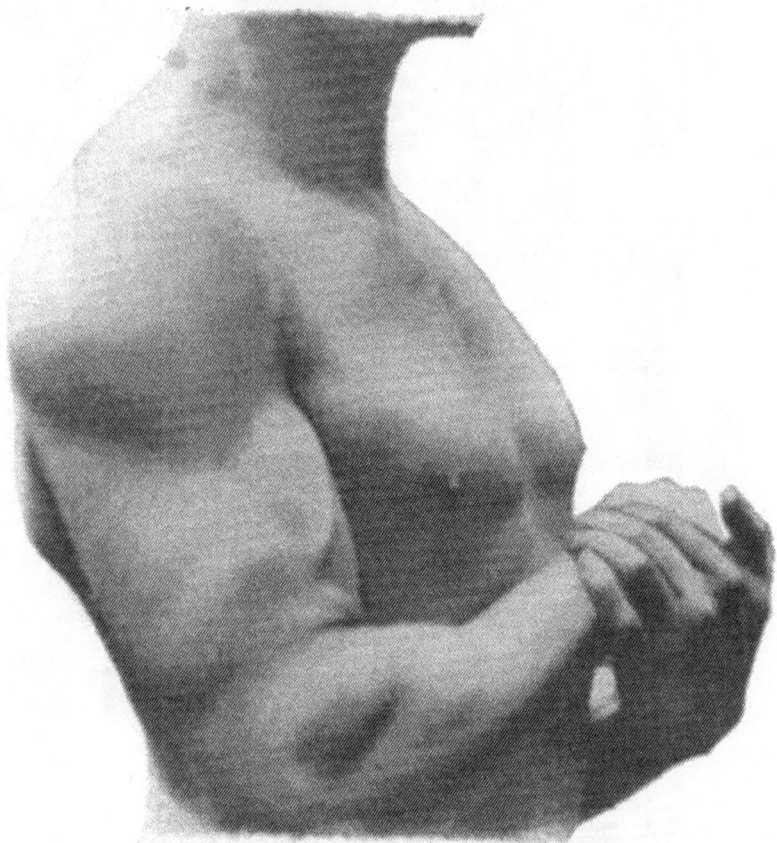

Photograph No. 19.

Exercise No. 11. Place left hand over back of right wrist and hand, as shown in illustration. Now, resisting movement slightly, bring the right forearm upward and outward from the right side. (See next photo.)

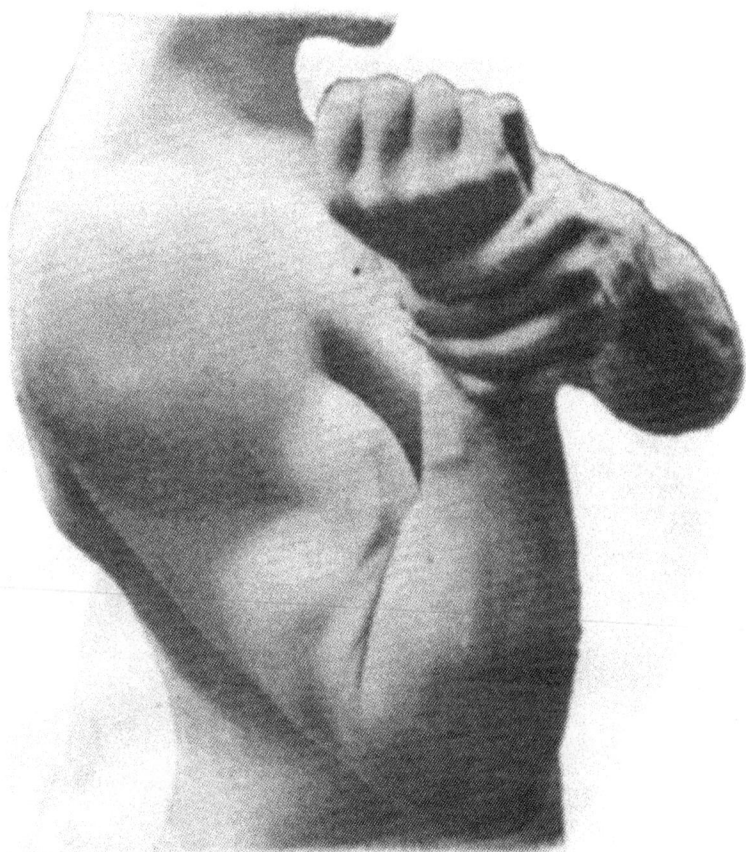

Photograph No. 20.

As far as possible, as shown in the above illustration. This is simply a twisting movement, the upper arm remaining stationary while the forearm is moved upward and outward. Take same exercise with the position of the arms and hands reversed. Continue the exercise with each arm until tired. For the muscles of the upper arm.

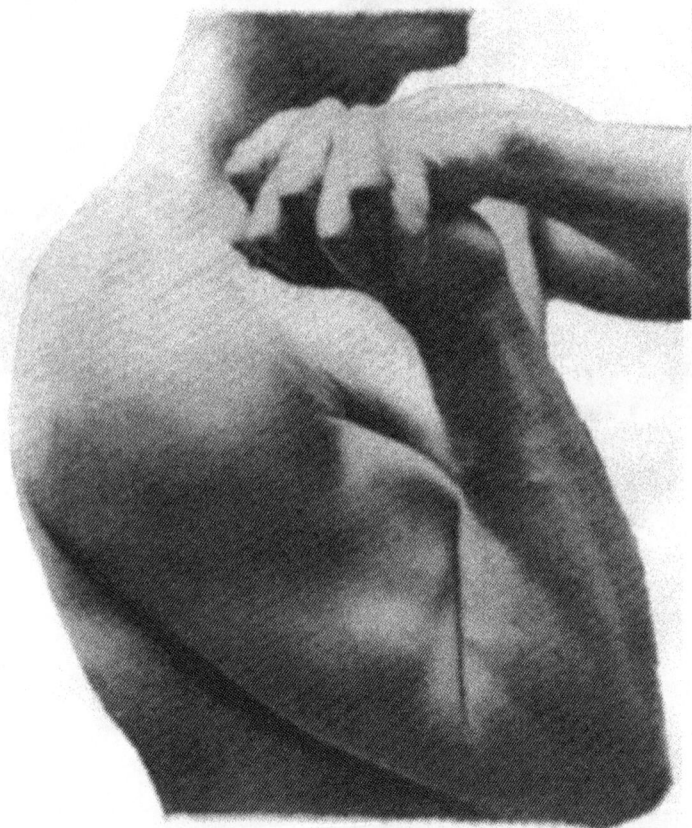

Photograph No. 21.

Exercise No. 12. Interlace fingers, as shown in above illustration. Now, resisting vigorously with the left hand, force the right hand over toward the left shoulder. (See next photo.)

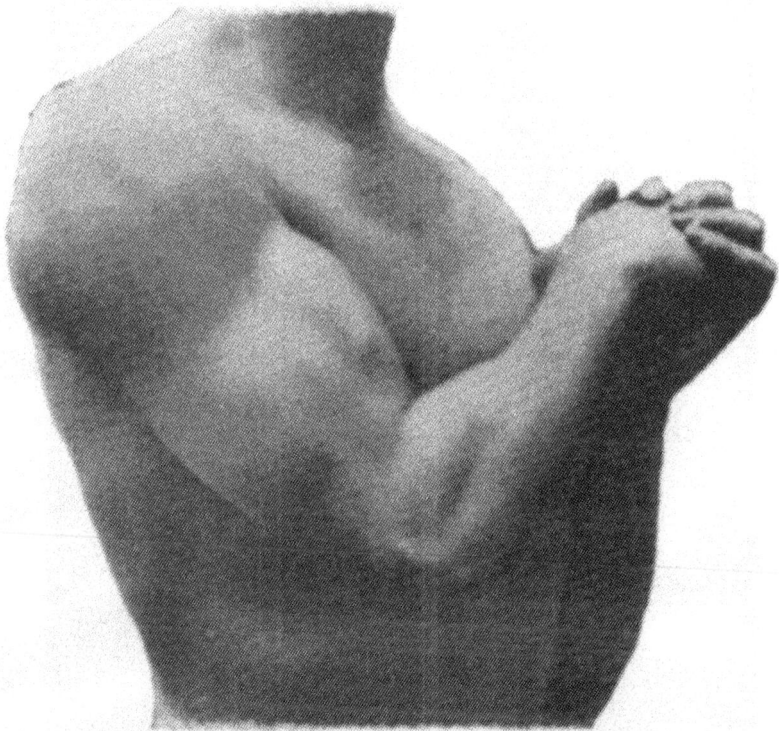

Photograph No. 22.

To position shown in illustration. You will note in this exercise that there is but little change in the bend of the arm at the elbow. Be sure to resist vigorously with the left hand. Take same exercise with the positions reversed and continue the exercise with each arm until tired. This is an excellent exercise to strengthen the muscles used in a contest where one tries to force down the arm of another.

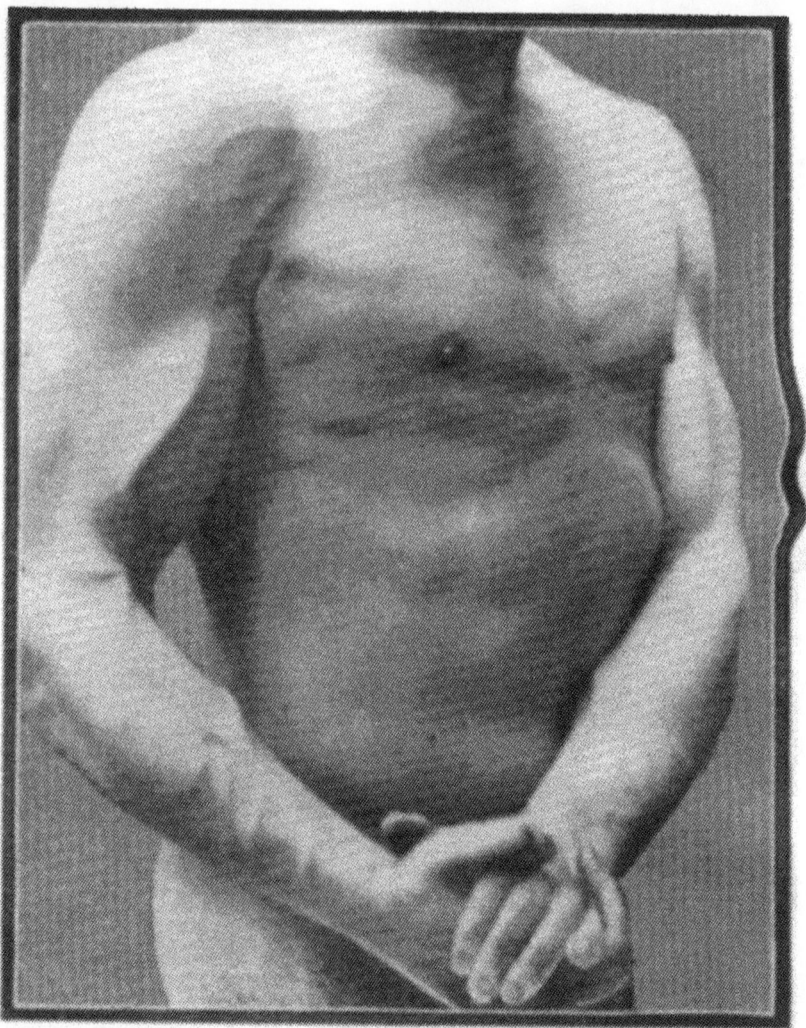

Photograph No. 23.

Exercise No. 13. Place the left hand in the right palm as shown in illustration. Now, resisting vigorously with the left arm, bend the right arm at the elbow, bringing the hand up as high as you can. (See next photo.)

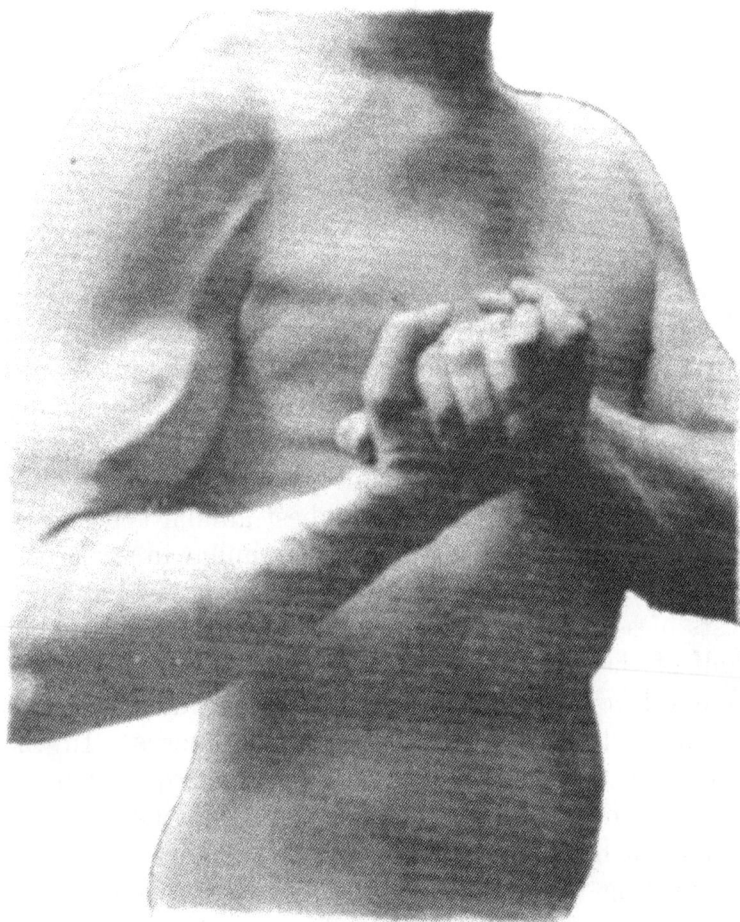

Photograph No. 24.

To the position shown in this illustration. The same exercise should be taken, placing the left hand over the back of the right hand. This slightly changes the action of the muscles used. Reverse the movement and take same exercise with other arm. This is another especially good exercise for the biceps of the upper arm.

CHAPTER XI.

ANATOMICAL STRUCTURE OF THE FOREARM.

We are assured by the evolutionists that man and the man-like ape are descended from common ancestors. We find that the latter, while possessing hands and arms that are closely allied to ours anatomically, uses all four of his limbs for locomotion, while man uses his legs only for the same purpose.

Nevertheless, even in the highest animal type, man, the arms and legs are wonderfully similar in structure. In the arm, the bony structure of the upper half consists of a single bone, called the humerus. The upper half of the leg is likewise a single shaft of bone, the femoral bone, which is constructed and attached in a manner almost identical with the humerus. In the lower leg there are two bones, attached by a wonderful system of hinge jointing. One of these is the principal bone, and the other serves as an auxiliary, permitting of more turning and twisting movements than are possible in the case of the upper leg.

It is the same with the forearm. There is almost the same kind of hinge joint, and in the lower arm we find two bones, the principal one being the ulna, while the smaller bone, which assists in and amplifies the movements of the limb, is known as the radius. This latter bone, the ulna, is termed the radial for the reason that it assists the forearm in turning, or radiating.

The bony structure of the forearm being so different

84

from that of the upper half of the limb, and being formed for the purpose of making possible a greater variety of movements, it follows that, in the forearm, we must look for a muscular structure totally different from that of the upper arm.   Indeed, the only point of similarity in the muscular structure of the two halves of the arm is, that the forearm as well as the upper arm, is supplied with muscles that flex the arm and muscles that extend it.

Let us, patiently and understandingly, look into the rather complex muscular arrangement that is encountered in the forearm.   I shall not weary you, my reader, with a discussion of minor muscles, and especially those that are deep below the surface.   It is sufficient for our present needs to comprehend the locations and uses of the more important muscles, and when the proper development of these has been assured, the requisite strengthening of the lesser muscles follows as a matter of course.

One of the powerful and much-used muscles of the forearm is the pronator radii teres.   Formidable as this name will seem to him who has not made some study of anatomy, the explanation of it is a simple one. Its name implies that it is a muscle used in the act of pronation, a term which I shall soon explain.   The second word of the name shows the connection of the muscle with the radius, or smaller bone of the forearm. And "teres" shows that this muscle formation is round and smooth.

Pronation may be explained in a few words.   Rest your entire forearm on a table with the back of the open hand downward.   Now, the hand and forearm are "supine."   In other words, the hand and forearm are resting in the position of "supination."   Now turn the hand over without lifting the elbow, so that the palm of the hand rests on the table. The wrist and lower part of the forearm will follow in the movement. This turning of the hand and wrist so that the palm lies downward is the act of "pronation." Hence a muscle that is employed in making this movement possible is called a pronator muscle. A muscle used in making an opposite movement that would lay the back of the hand on the table is called a supinator muscle. It is not necessary, however, to rest the hand and forearm on a table or other surface. The acts of pronation and supination are performed by their guiding muscles in an almost endless variety of movements in every possible position of the arm.

The pronator radii teres might well be compared with the biceps of the upper arm, for this pronator is a two-headed muscle and has its insertion in a single tendon. One head of the pronator arises from the humerus, or upper arm bone, just above the jointing with the ulna and from the tendon that passes over the inside of the elbow and is the common origin of the other muscles. It also arises from the fascia, or sheath, over the muscles of the upper forearm. The second head of this muscle is a thin bundle of fibres which arises from the lower end of the humerus, and this second head joins the first at an acute angle. It is between these two heads that the important median nerve enters the forearm. The muscle passes slantingly across the forearm, and the insertion is in an impression at the middle of the outer surface of the radius. The insertion of the biceps muscle is under this pronator muscle.

Just inside of this pronator muscle, and on the little finger side of the forearm, is the flexor carpi radialis.

This name is not hard to understand. "Flexor" shows the use of the muscle; "carpi" indicates that the muscle is employed in flexing the carpus, as the collection of wrist bones is termed, and "radialis" shows the connection with the radius, or smaller bone of the forearm. It arises from the inner condyle, or lower end of the humerus, passes down over the front of the forearm in a course somewhat less oblique than that of the pronator, and the insertion is by a tendon that is attached to the metacarpal (back-of-the-hand) bone of the forefinger.

Of the palmaris longus no more need be said than that it has its origin near the source of the flexor carpi radialis, and that it is still further to the inside of the forearm, the insertion being in the palmar fascia—the sheath that covers the muscles of the palm of the hand. The palmaris longus should be well developed as an aid to gripping strongly. But this muscle is an uncertain one; it is subject to many variations, and in some instances is altogether absent.

The flexor carpi ulnaris lies along the exact side of the front of the forearm. It is bicipital—that is, like the biceps of the upper arm, it has two heads. One of these heads arises from the inner condyle of the humerus, this condyle being the inner of the two projections of the lower end of the humerus that fit into the sockets at the upper ends of the ulna and radius. The other head arises from the olecranon process—or "funny-bone"—of the ulna. The insertion is close to the inner side of the hand.

The supinator longus is the largest muscle of the forearm, and it is the nearest to the surface. In general it may be said that its course is along the outer, or thumb side of the forearm. This muscle is sometimes called the brachio-radialis. It is a fleshy muscle for the upper two-thirds of its course, and in the latter third of its course it takes on, as it progresses, more and more of the nature of a tendon. While exercising the arm, this muscle and its tendon can be felt very plainly. This muscle should stand out hard and firm when the arm is tensed or in motion. As the purpose of this muscle is to supply the action of supination, its work is felt most effectively when the hand and forearm are rested on a table, palm downward—or pronate—and then the hand and lower forearm are turned over in the act of supination, so that the back of the hand rests on the table. This experiment, when made with the arm well tensed, should show a very hard, knotted muscle—or else its development is not what it should be.

This supinator longus muscle arises principally from the lower end of the humerus. The insertion is by a tendon near the base of the radius.

Of the muscles of the back of the forearm, I wish to call your attention first to the extensor carpi ulnaris, for this muscle plays a very big part in the work of straightening—or "extending"—the forearm after it has been flexed. Its movements are observed readily during any vigorous action that extends the forearm. This muscle is found to begin at the elbow, and runs along the back of the forearm on the little finger side. It is a broad, tough muscle that bulges a great deal in tensed movements of the powerful forearm. It arises principally from the lower end of the humerus, and from other points, among them, the strong muscular fascia of the forearm. The insertion is by means of a tendon at the base of the metacarpal (back-of-the-hand) bone of the little finger.

The extensor communis digitorum—which means simply that this muscle is of the extensor kind and affects the fingers in common—is found in the center of the back of the forearm. This is another very important muscle of this part of the forearm. It arises, as the other muscles do, from the lower end of the humerus; by an arrangement of tendons this muscle passes over the back of the hand, and the tendinous branches are inserted at the bases of the four fingers. The movements of these tendons can be felt by closing and opening the hand strongly, and by employing the other hand in moving over the back of its fellow.

CHAPTER XII.

So numerous and diverse are the movements of which the forearm is capable that it is possible to devise almost innumerable exercises that will be of great benefit in building it up. In general it may be said that any exercise is good for the forearm which gives it strong and vigorous work. The exercises that I present herewith are those that I advise as the best possible.

Bear in mind, always, that it is of very little use to try to be an all-around athlete unless the forearm is splendidly trained and developed. In almost any form of exercise you are doomed to failure if you have not succeeded in building up forearms that fully meet the demands of a high strandard of power. Do not, therefore, reserve these exercises for occasional and indifferent use, but keep at them systematically and industriously. Strong forearms will aid you greatly in strengthening many other portions of the body. And the muscles of the forearms increase in size very rapidly under good training. This is one of the parts of the human frame where encouraging results, due to proper exercises, are noted most quickly.

The first exercise for the forearm, number fourteen, as shown in photograph 25, gives the preliminary work in the task of strengthening the forearm in

90

general, and those muscles that are used most in gripping, in particular. The wrist shares extensively in this work. Right here I wish to tell my readers that weak wrists are altogether too common among Americans. Comparatively few men, in training, give much attention to the wrists. Those who do not do so, make a huge mistake.

Exercise number fifteen, as shown by the next two photographs, serves to continue the good work begun by the preceding exercise. Yet it has been my experience that many students of physical training do not appear to realize just how hard the pressure with the resisting hand should be made. Put in *all* the resistance reasonably possible with the left hand, using force enough with the right to overcome the resistance. In resisting with the right hand against the left, give the left hand all the resistance that it is possible for it to overcome. Exercise number sixteen, explained graphically by two photographs, gives the same kind of work for the wrists, at the same time vigorously employing some of the other muscles of the forearm more effectively.

This last work is practically reversed in exercise number seventeen. It will be noticed, by the way, that throughout I have made it a point, as far as is possible, to have one exercise followed by another that is its opposite. Every muscle in the body is resisted by some other muscle, and this alternate work employs one muscle against its opposite to the best advantage. If you keep to the exercises in the order in which I have given them you will find that you are reaping the best results from them.

Exercise number eighteen, gives a form of wrist and forearm work that employs the muscles in a still differ-

ent fashion.   While you are exercising, remember what
I said about the muscles in the last chapter, and study
to see just what muscles you are now employing, and
try to understand why you are benefiting such muscles.
This ability to analyze the nature and benefits of an
exercise will come to you very readily after a little
practice with your reasoning faculties.   And you will
find that it makes your exercising more enjoyable, too,
and also renders it possible to get more benefit by knowing just how much of each exercise to take in order to
secure the utmost all-around development in your individual case.

Exercises number nineteen and twenty are explained
by photographs 34, 35, 36 and 37.   Here, again, varying uses of different muscles are made in the most
effective manner.   In all of them the wrist shares, as
it should, in the development that is given to the
forearm in order that the work performed by the lower
arm may be harmonious throughout.

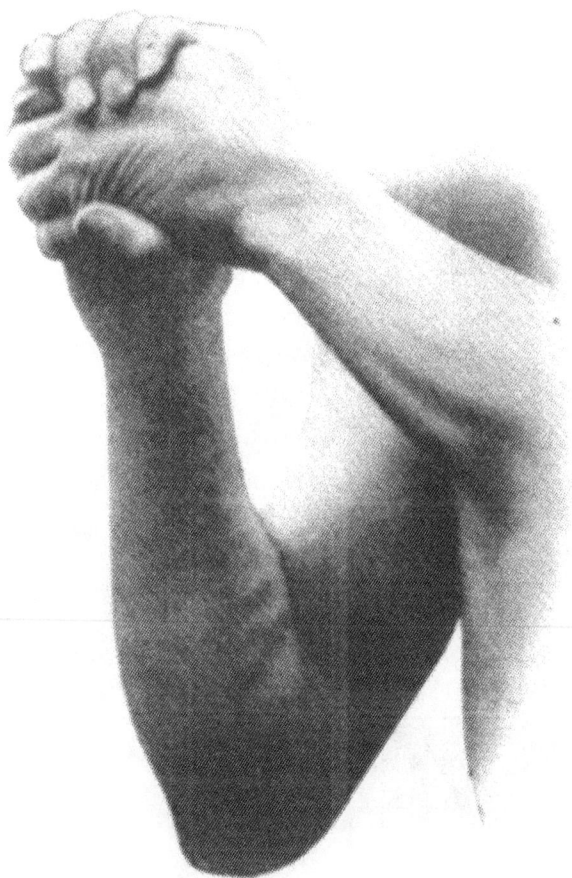

Photograph No. 25.

Exercise No. 14. This exercise consists simply of gripping the hands as tightly as possible, as shown in the illustration. First grip right hand with left, and then left with right, alternating from one to the other. Continue the exercise until the gripping muscles of the forearm are thoroughly tired.

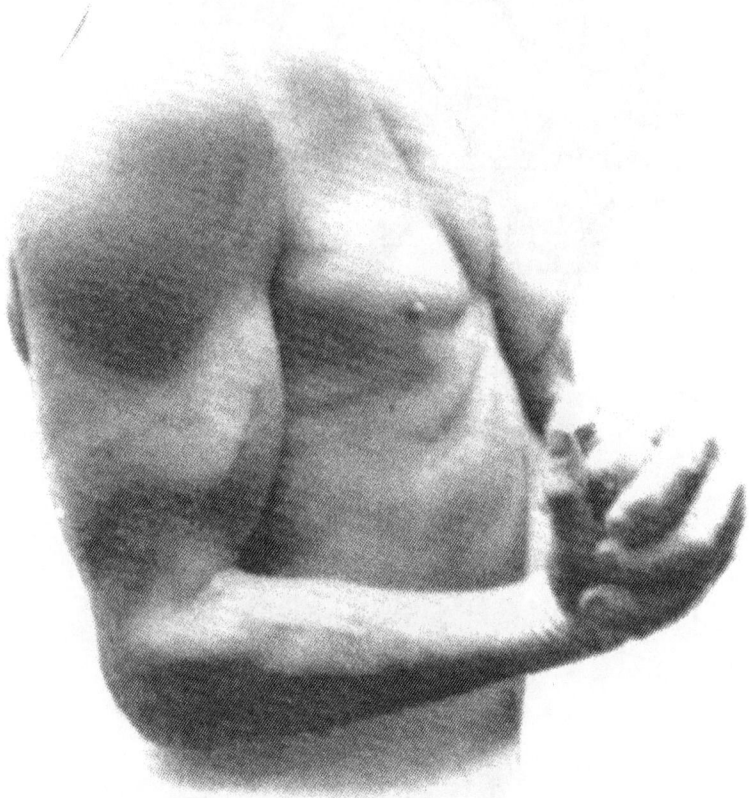

Photograph No. 26.

Exercise No. 15. Hold the arm in the position shown in illustration with the wrist bent and twisted over far to the right. Now, pressing vigorously against movement with your left hand, twist the right wrist inward as far as you can. (See next photo.)

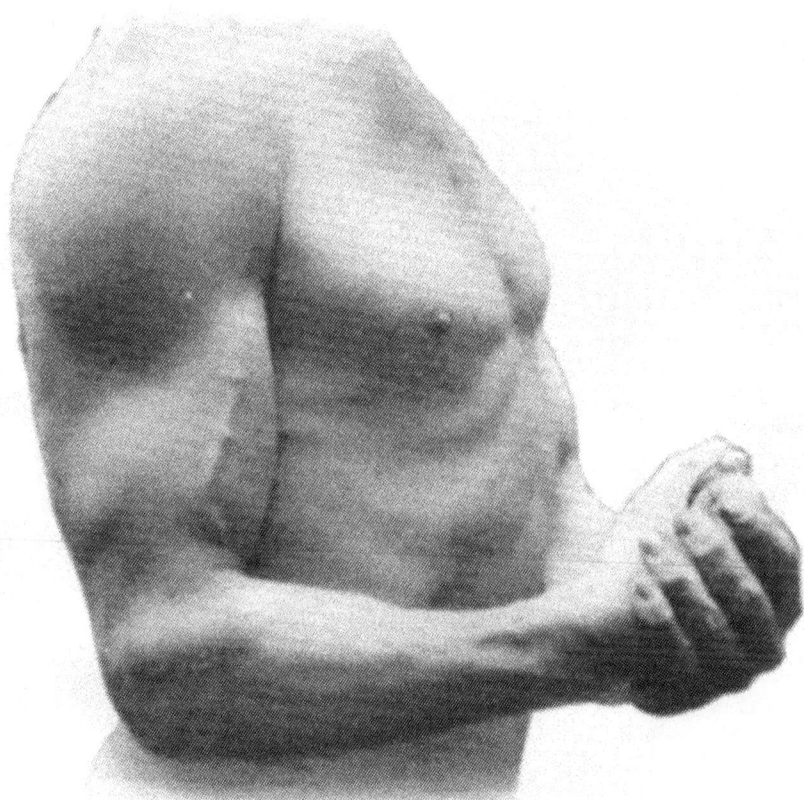

Photograph No. 27.

To position shown in above illustration. Take same exercise with the position of the hands reversed. Continue the exercise until tired, and be careful to keep the wrist bent as far as possible during the entire movement.

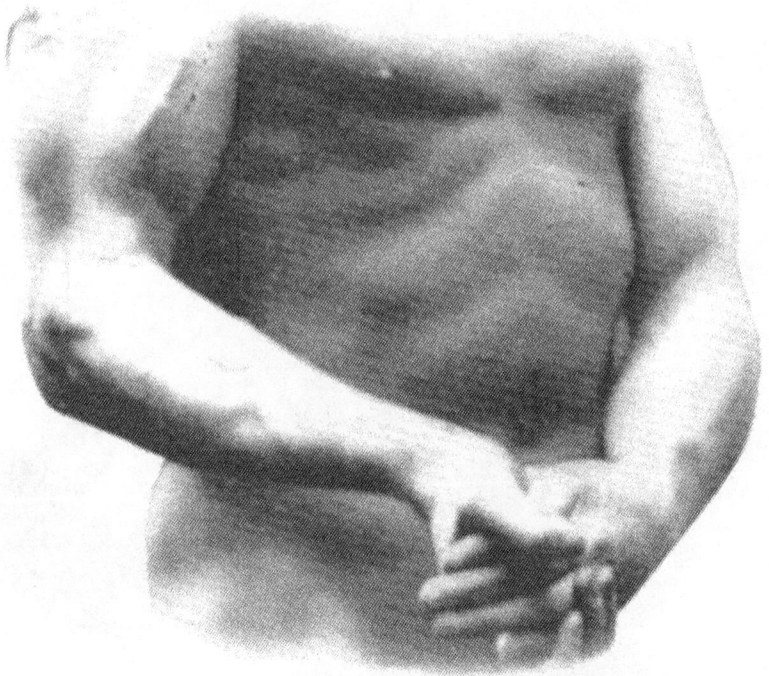

Photograph No. 28.

Exercise No. 16. Place left hand in the right palm as shown in illustration. Now, resisting the movement with the left hand, bend right wrist and force the hand upward. (See next photo.)

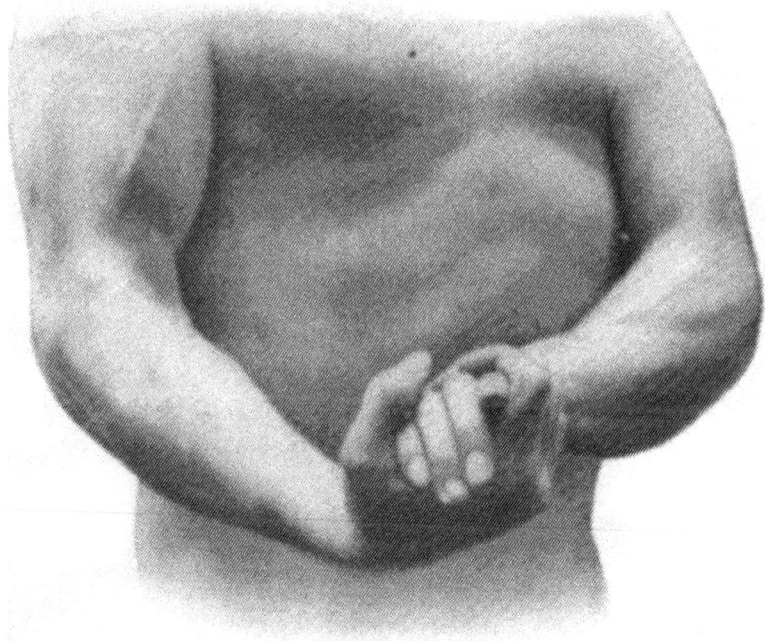

Photograph No. 29.

To the position shown in the above illustration. Take same exercise with the position of the hands reversed. Continue the exercise until the muscles of the front part of the forearm are tired.

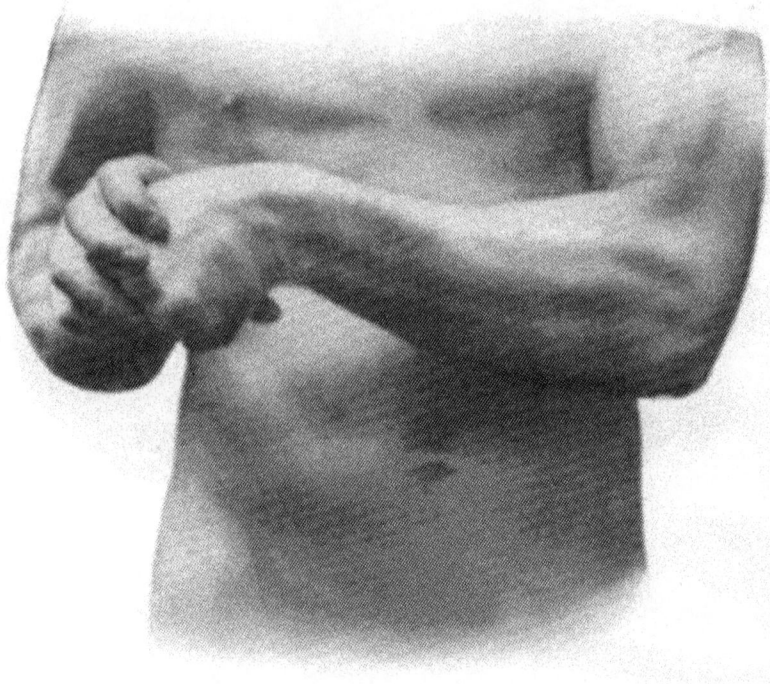

Photograph No. 30.

Exercise No. 17. Grasp the left hand with the wrist bent
s shown in illustration. Now, resisting the movement with
the right hand, straighten the left wrist, forcing the hand upward
as far as possible. (See next photo.)

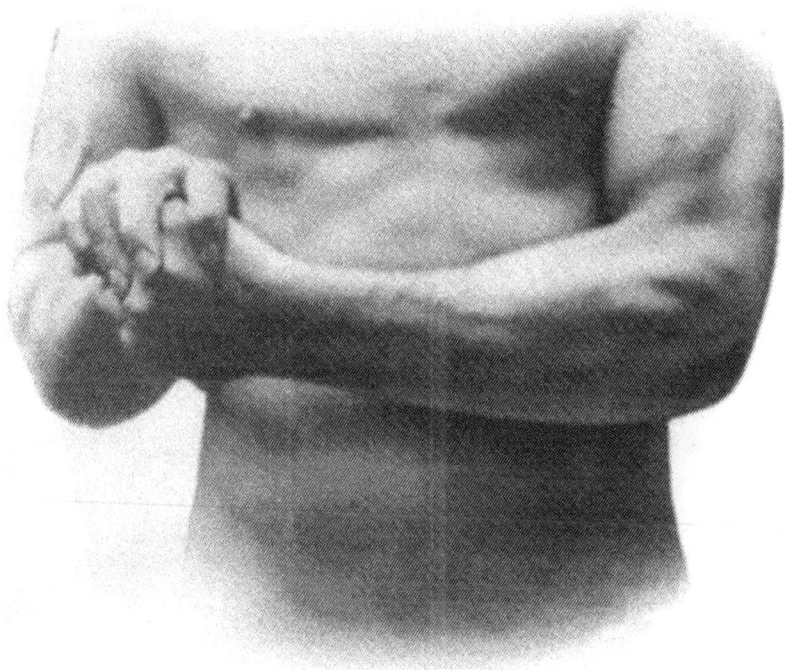

Photograph No. 31.

To the position shown in the above illustration. Take same exercise with the position of the hands reversed. Continue until the muscles on the side of the forearm tire.

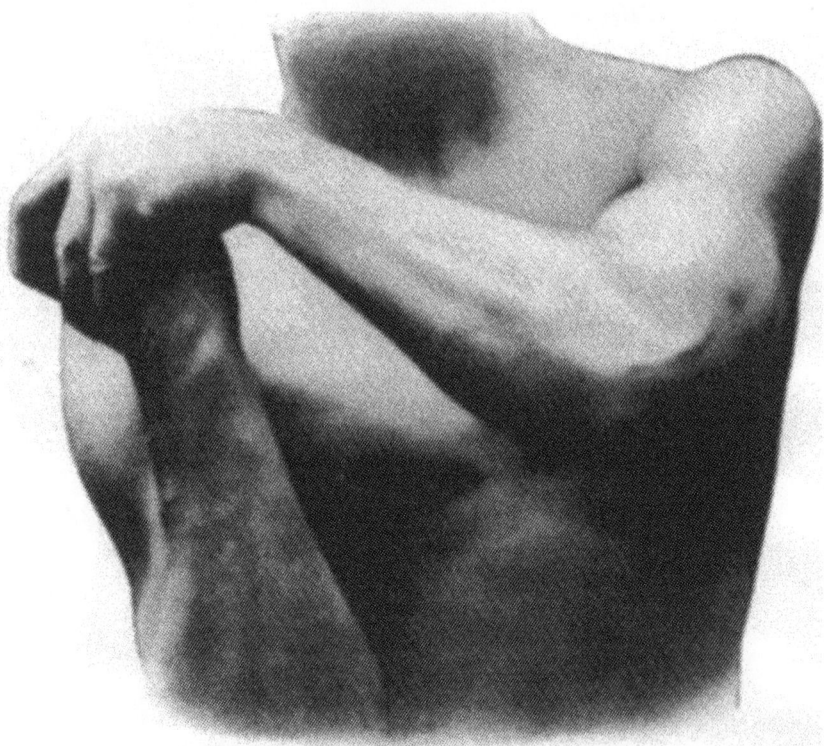

Photograph No. 32.

Exercise No. 18. Grasp right wrist with left hand, with the wrist bent as far over to the right as possible. Now, resisting the movement with the left arm, bend the wrist inward and toward the left shoulder as far as you possibly can. (See next photo.)

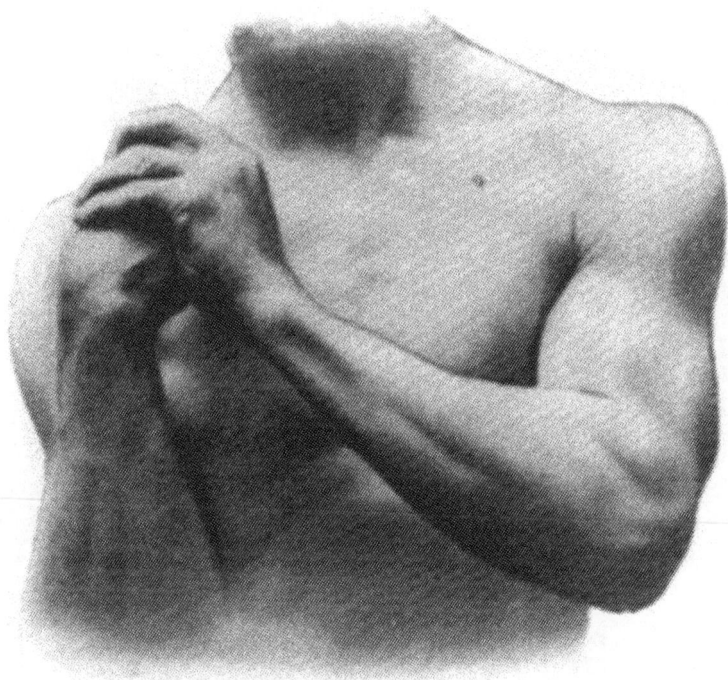

Photograph No. 33.

To the position shown in the above illustration. Take the same exercise with the position of the hands reversed, and continue with each until the muscles are tired.

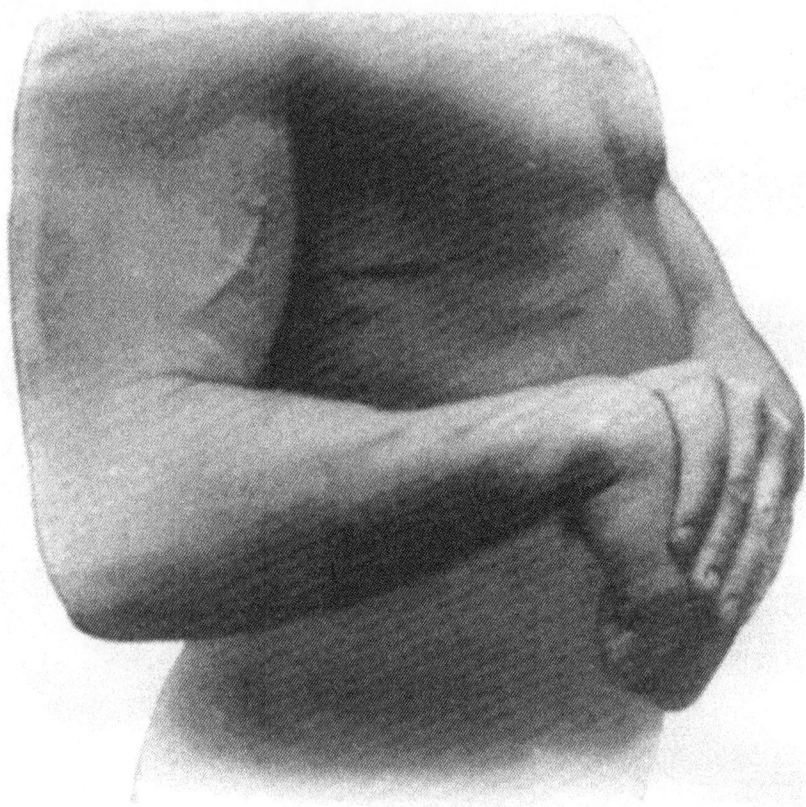

Photograph No. 34.

Exercise No. 19. Place the left thumb under the right wrist
and the fingers of the left hand over the right, as shown in illustration.   Now, pressing against the movement vigorously, bend
wrist, (See next photo.)

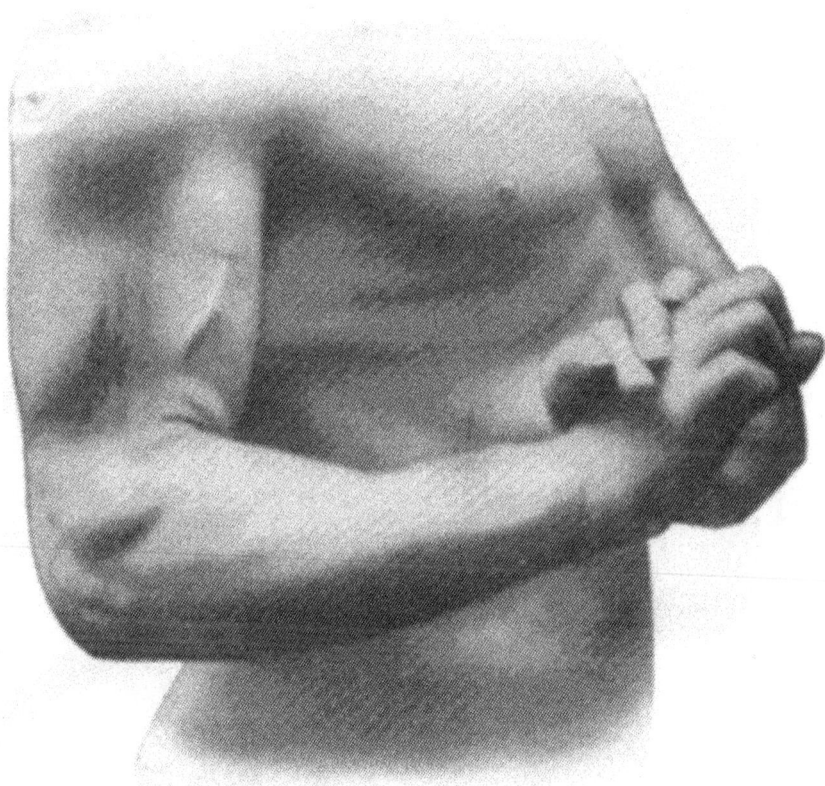

Photograph No. 35.

To position shown in above illustration. Continue movement until muscles tire. Same exercise with the position of the hands reversed. This exercise is excellent for developing the muscles on the back of the forearm.

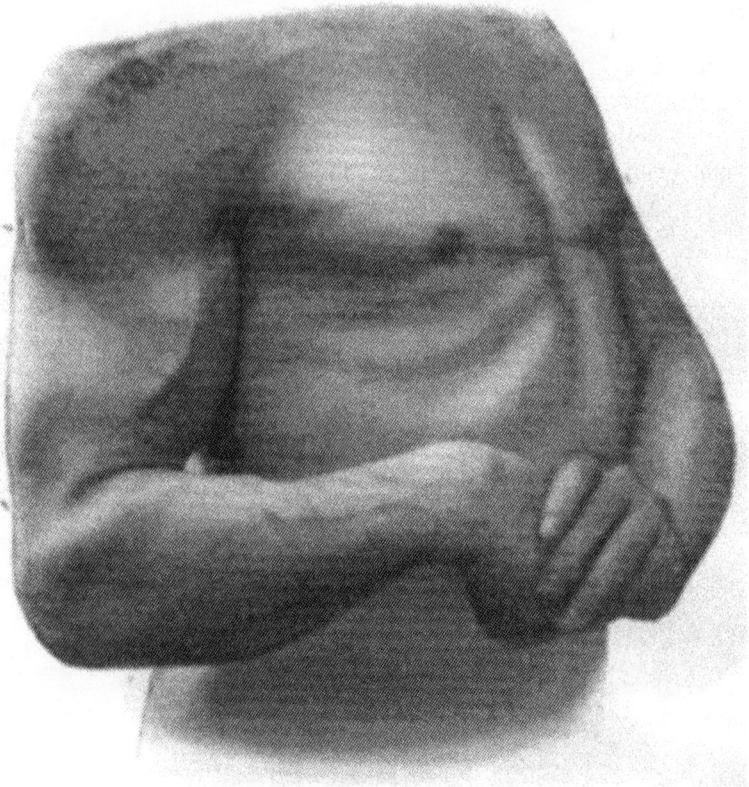

Photograph No. 36.

Exercise No. 20. Begin with the wrist of the right hand bent inward as far as possible, and turned far over as shown in the illustration. Now, place the left hand on the right, and resisting the movement considerably twist the forearm and turn the wrist upward, (See next photo.)

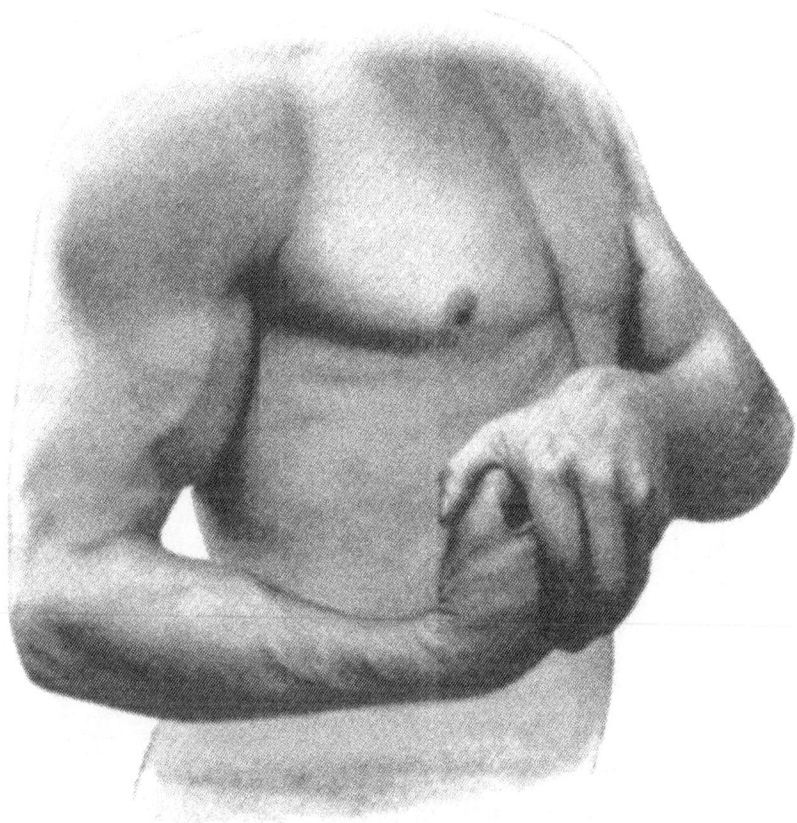

Photograph No. 37.

As shown in above illustration. Continue movement until muscles tire. Same exercise with position of the hands reversed. This exercise develops the muscles of the forearm, and also a small muscle of the upper arms.

CHAPTER XIII.

Exercises for Strengthening the Fingers.

It would be a strange anomaly of training, indeed, if one were to give much thought to the strengthening of the forearms, and yet pay scant attention to increasing the muscular powers of the fingers. For it is through the fingers that most of the work of the forearms is performed.

It is true, too, that all of the work undertaken to the end of securing great power in the fingers will be reflected in added strength of the forearms; but it is not necessarily true that the tasks of strengthening the forearm will result in direct benefit to the fingers. For this reason, special exercises must be designed for bringing the fingers up to their utmost capacity for strength.

As in the case of the forearms, the fingers respond with surprising rapidity to wisely directed exercise. After a fortnight, even, of proper exercise, the novitiate in physical training is surprised at the greatly increased amount of strength in his fingers.

What are the tasks in which the fingers are most severely employed? The answer to this question, combined with a little thought, will furnish the student with infallible hints as to the best methods of exercise. It is a self-evident proposition that any given muscle may be trained best through the use of some exercise that closely resembles the work which the muscle is called upon to naturally perform—with this difference only, that the exercise should call for more exertion than would the natural work of the muscle.

What are the important kinds of work that man is usually called upon to perform with his fingers? Gripping and holding mainly. Sometimes it is necessary to press with the fingers, either point-on, or with the backs or the insides of the fingers. When, on the other hand, the fist is clenched, all muscular energy for a blow must be furnished by the forearm, the upper arm, the shoulder, and so on, and in a lesser degree by a large array of muscles, including even those of the calf.

Exercise number twenty-one is adapted to the purpose of finger developing. It trains the muscles for pressing the fingers forcefully, but it also adds greatly to the power of the muscles used in gripping. There is also the advantage that each finger is trained in the work of contending against other muscles.

And this work furnishes an excellent test for the gradually growing strength of the fingers. I have advised that the exercise be continued until the fingers are tired. Note how long it takes you to tire the fingers at the outset, and then observe, from week to week, just how much longer you are able to continue the work before your fingers become fatigued. The increase in strength will be in due ratio to the increased length of time that you can continue the exercise.

This applies too, to exercise number twenty-two, as shown in photographs 40 and 41. This exercise will prove a little more difficult, and fatigue is likely to result sooner than in the case of the preceding exercise, but for this reason, all the more effort should be made to acquire the strength necessary to do the work without tiring at too early a stage.

Exercise twenty-three has the advantage of giving the thumbs a task along with the fingers. As each thumb is employed in connection with four different fingers, the thumbs come in for a very excellent share of needful effort. The thumbs should be given a great deal of work against the fingers, the latter overcoming the thumbs only by the performance of the hardest kind of work. The thumbs are naturally more powerful than any of the fingers, and if they are given hard enough work their supremacy over the fingers will be maintained throughout.

Naturally any form of work, exercise or stunt which taxes the fingers will serve to strengthen them. You may have noted that manual workers who are accustomed to handle heavy objects with their hands and fingers—bricklayers, for instance—invariably have very hard and strong, and usually large fingers, and although these may be somewhat the result of inheritance, yet the work they do unquestionably does tend to strengthen and even enlarge them. The truth of this would be evident if their fingers were compared with those of light occupations, book-keepers, for instance. Remember, however, that it is possible to greatly strengthen the fingers with but a very slight increase in their size.

One commonly practiced method of strengthening the fingers is the lifting of weights with each finger separately, each day lifting as heavy a weight as the finger will stand, and gradually increasing the weights as the strength of the fingers grows. As a result some remarkable finger-lifting records have been made. Another method is to press down with each finger on an ordinary scale, each day ascertaining at how many pounds the balance can be tipped. These might of course be resorted to occasionally as a help in the strengthening of your fingers, though they might prove too great a strain and really are not to be advised so much as the free movement resisting exercises illustrated herewith. You might, however, use a scale in this manner once in a while merely as a test of strength to show what your improvement has been.

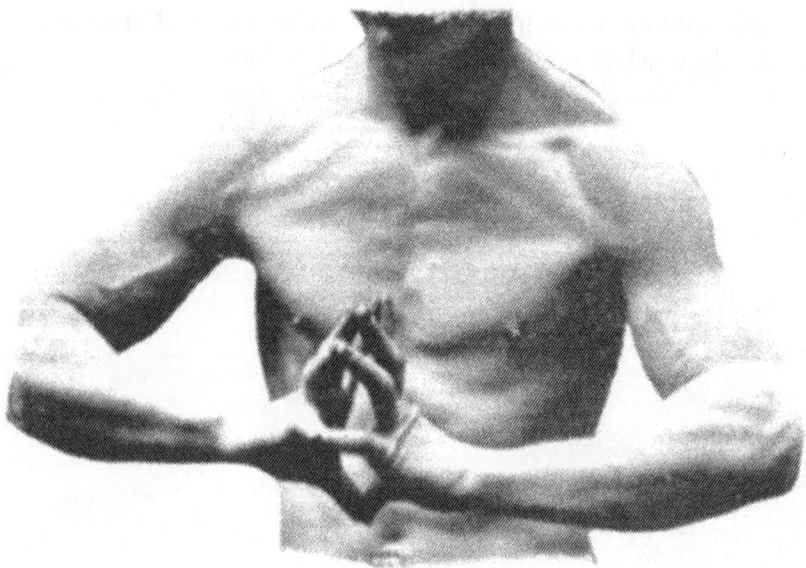

Photograph No. 38.

Exercise No. 21. Place the fingers together as shown in illustration. While pressing them together with the strength of the arms, straighten the fingers and force them. (See next photo.)

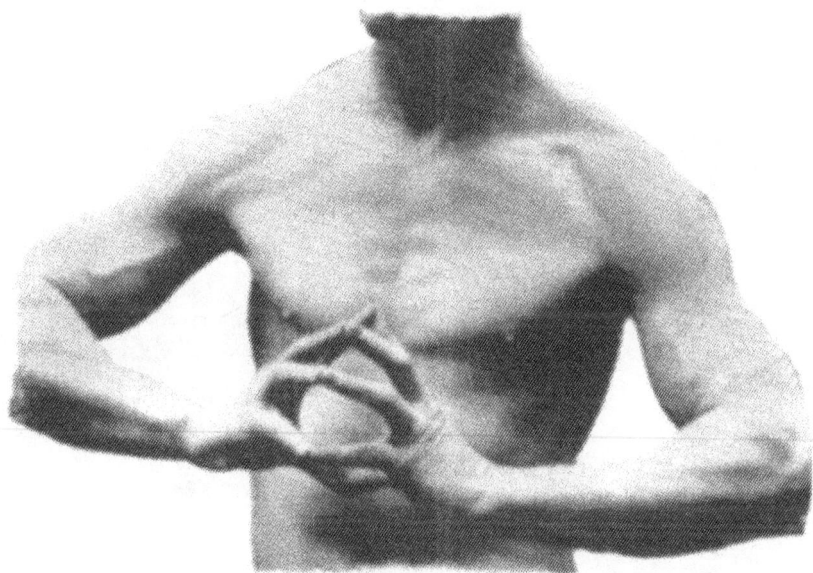

Photograph No. 39.

To the position shown in this photograph. Continue the exercise until the fingers tire. This exercise is specially beneficial for strengthening the fingers and developing the gripping power. Each finger is required to make an individual effort, and this exercise alone will usually be found far superior to the ordinary grip machine for increasing the strength of your fingers and wrists.

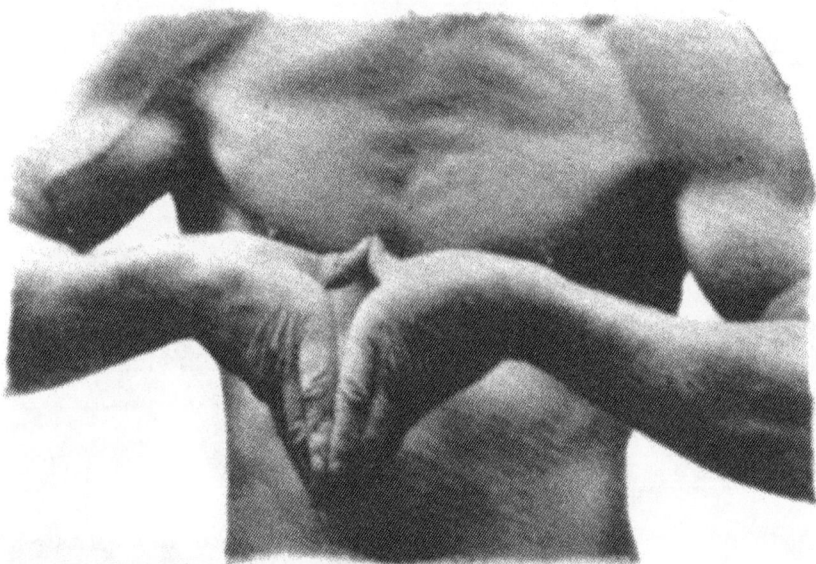

Photograph No. 40.

Exercise No. 22. Place the fingers together as shown in this illustration. Now press them together strongly with the strength of the arms, and slowly roll the ends of the fingers and the thumb until they are in position shown in the next illustration.

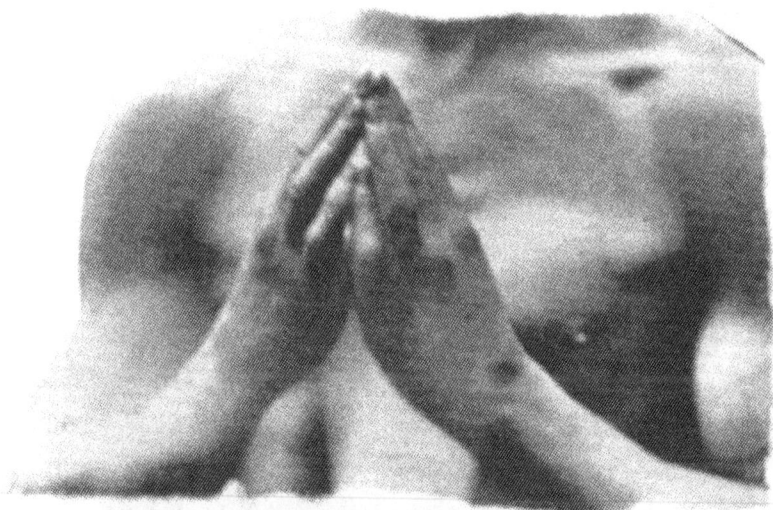

Photograph No. 41.

This may be found rather difficult the first few attempts, but practice will soon enable you to easily perform it. If this exercise is taken properly it exerts the fingers in both side movements. Continue the exercise until the fingers tire. This exercise will be found valuable for increasing the strength of the fingers.

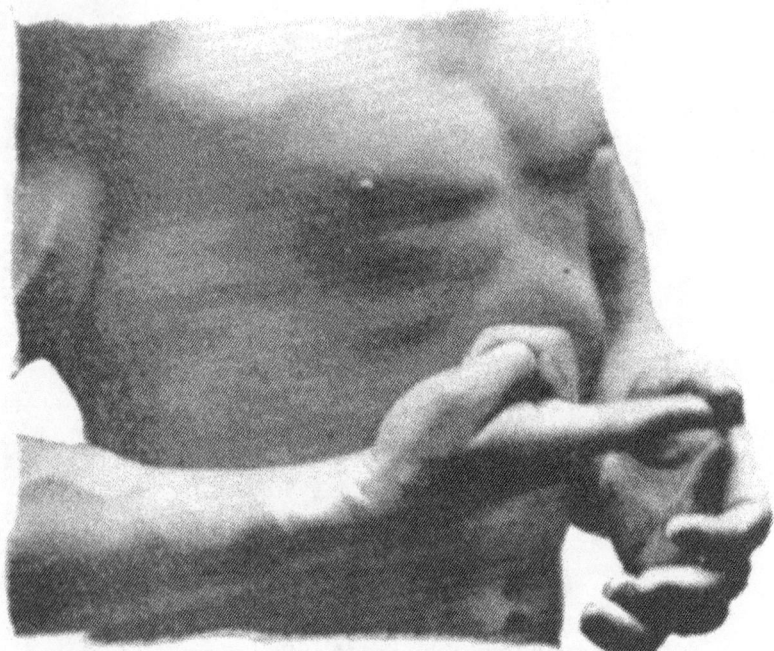

Photograph No. 42.

Exercise No. 23. Place the thumb of the left hand on the first finger of the right hand as shown in the illustration. Now, pressing slightly against the movement of the left thumb, bend the first right finger. (See next photo.)

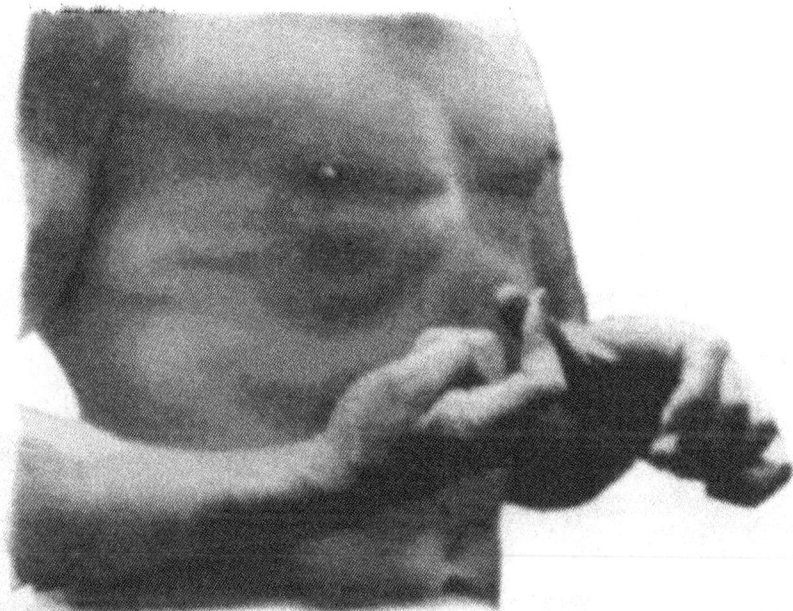

Photograph No. 43.

To position shown in illustration. Continue the movement until the finger tires. Each of the fingers and the thumbs of both hands can be exercised in a similar manner, if one is specially anxious to strengthen all the fingers to the greatest possible extent. For those who are desirous of possessing a steel-like grip and for those who are suffering with writer's cramp, these exercises will be found specially beneficial.

CHAPTER XIV.

ANATOMICAL STRUCTURE OF THE MUSCLES OF THE NECK.

It is all but superfluous to point out why great strength in the neck is so very much to be desired. All of us instinctively associate neck strength with remarkable general muscular power. Whether in the case of the prize-fighter, or of the laborer, we look for what we call the "bull neck." If we find this set on a pair of massive shoulders we naturally look for strength out of the ordinary on the part of the owner of the neck.

In the neck of an ox we find the muscles standing out in strong relief when that animal is hauling a burden of unusual weight. In the tiger, we find the longer neck, more supple, lithe and slender, yet withal a neck of immense power. It is this latter type of neck that is better suited to the athlete than is the short, sturdy neck of the ox.

In all feats of strength where the strain is distributed with some approach to evenness over the entire body, the neck comes in for its full share of hard work. It follows that if the neck muscles be weak the athlete is vitally defective in his physical make-up.

And there is still another reason than the need of meeting mere muscular demands why the neck should be powerful. The best development of all the functions of the body depends upon the nourishment—in other words, the building up—of the brain. Now health and vigor of the brain are dependent on the nourishment that the blood derives from properly digested food in the stomach and intestines. If the brain be not fed plentifully and richly, its structure is bound to deteriorate. Ample feeding of the brain by healthy blood quickens and invigorates all the faculties and the bodily activities that spring from them.

Enough attention to the muscular development of the neck increases the size of all of its parts. But the muscles of the neck are by no means alone in sharing in the benefits that arise from their development. As the neck is increased in size, there is more room for the great blood vessels that enter the head through the neck to grow and so allow of the blood flowing more copiously to and from the brain. This does not mean any added danger of a "rush of blood to the brain," for, while the enlarged arteries carry an increased quantity, the enlarged veins bring it away again as promptly, and so the balance of the flow of the blood is maintained. But exercise quickens the flow of blood to the brain, and, from physiological causes of an obvious nature, carries a better quality there at the same time. Thus the brain is benefited directly by strict attention to the muscular development of the neck.

Then the nerves, those vassals yet allies of the brain, must come in for their share of the incidental benefit. Every muscle in the body is controlled by directing nerves. Without "orders" from a nerve, no muscle is capable of action. Small wonder, then, that physical trainers of to-day give the strictest heed to the nervous condition of those in their charge. An athlete with poor nerves is a pitiable sort of athlete indeed! Yet the proper muscular development of the neck will result in a better, truer condition of the nerves, and render the athlete stronger and more competent in every member of his bodily system.

The muscles in the neck are many and varied in their purposes. Only a few need be discussed, for these are easily found and their strength tested and, if these muscles be properly exercised, the other neck muscles will become strengthened as a matter of course.

In the front and at the sides of the neck we have the platysma myoides muscle. This is a very broad and somewhat thin sheet of muscle, which proper exercise of the neck will do much to strengthen and thicken. I shall not attempt to give all of the points of origin and insertion of this muscle, as to do so would be confusing my reader with a needlessly bewildering array of anatomical data. It is enough to say that the upper portion of this muscle is found covering the chin and jaw, and it extends downward, enveloping the whole of the front of the neck. The muscle covers also the sides of the neck, and extends down over the collar bone and the shoulder. It is the action of this myoides muscle that causes the wrinkling of the skin of the neck when the latter is brought into extreme muscular action. This muscle serves also to protect the great carotid artery, and the jugular vein as well.

The various uses of this muscle are too numerous to be given in detail. But it may be said that it draws down the jaw, lowers the under lip, and in many ways affects the expression of the features. Beneath it there is a fascia, or sheathing of muscle, that surrounds the neck, and the strength of this fascia (the deep cervical fascia, it is called) is developed by precisely the same work that strengthens and toughens the platysma myoides.

That muscle of the neck which is most readily found,

and which is capable of the most visible development, is known as the sterno-cleido-mastoid. It is found just back of the lobe of the ear, crosses the front of the neck obliquely, and continues down to the breast-bone. In many respects this is the most important muscle of the neck, as it is certainly the most powerful. When the neck muscles are tensed, the sterno-cleido-mastoid should stand out very distinctly to the vision. To the finger tips it will feel like a strong, quivering rope.

The origin of this muscle is in two heads. One arises from the upper portion of the breast bone, and the other from the collar bone. At the heads this muscle is separated in its parts, but these gradually merge, and they are completely joined at about the middle of the neck. The insertion of this muscle is at the mastoid process behind the ear.

In action the sterno-cleido-mastoid muscle serves many purposes. When only the muscle on one side of the neck is employed it draws the head over to the shoulder on that side. Another movement of the muscle rotates the head so as to turn the face to the shoulder on the other side. It is in this motion that its movement is felt very plainly. If, however, the head be fixed in position, and not moved, the sterno-cleido-mastoid muscles on both sides are employed together in raising the chest in the act of forced inspiration of breath.

At the sides of the back of the neck and extending out over the shoulders is the trapezius muscle. This is really a muscle of the back, and will be mentioned again when I come to the consideration of the back muscles. But it is much benefited by all proper neck work.

Anatomically, the splenius muscle, also, is described

as one of the muscles of the back, but it plays so important a part in the work of the neck that I shall say a few words about it here. The splenius may be felt in the tensed neck just back of the sterno-cleido-mastoid. It runs obliquely up and forward. It begins in the upper portion of the back and ends in the neck.

This splenius is a broad, flat muscle, of considerable toughness. As it ascends into the neck it divides into two portions, one of which is known as the splenius capitis and the other as the splenius colli. The capitis is inserted mainly at the mastoid process, and the colli into the two or three upper vertebræ of the neck. These splenius muscles are employed in drawing the head directly backward; they aid also in drawing the head to one side, and somewhat in rotating it. Most important of all of the functions of the splenius muscle is to keep the head in an erect position.

CHAPTER XV.

EXERCISES FOR DEVELOPING THE MUSCLES OF THE NECK.

As I explained in the last chapter, the proper development of the muscles of the neck is a subject of the greatest importance to the athlete. Not only is the structure of the neck improved but the functional and muscular tone of the body is also directly and beneficially affected.

And the head is capable of so many motions, and the neck is subject to so many different forms of strain, that a considerable variety of exercises is needed, but those that I have given herein are the most valuable and sufficient in scope to meet all needs.

The range of neck work is illustrated by the photographs numbered from 44 to 53. It would be hard, indeed, to pick out any one of these exercises as being more important than any of the others in the set. All of them should be industriously and vigorously gone through with at one bout of exercise. Do not stop this neck work until the muscles of the region are comfortably tired.

As you proceed, watch the effect upon your muscles of each of these exercises. If you are observant, you will gain the most valuable kind of information as to the muscular needs of your neck. You will find, of course, that some of the exercises tire you more quickly than do others. Exercise twenty-six will be found

to be considerably more fatiguing than twenty-four.
After a few practice bouts, covering, say, a week or ten
days, you should find that you are able to do
number twenty-six with less fatigue than you did
number twenty-four. At the end of the second week
of practice you should certainly be able to do twice as
much of the neck work in a single exercise bout as you
did in the first week, and this ratio of improvement
should continue for some weeks, before you begin to
find yourself approaching a somewhat definite limit of
endurance in regard to these exercises.

After you have been giving a portion of your attention daily for, say, three or four weeks to this work, it
will be well to occasionally test your increased neck
power by subjecting the muscles involved to more
and more severe strains.

Try choking yourself, for instance, and note how
much pressure of the fingers you can stand at the
throat, saving yourself from strangling by tensing the
neck muscles and "throwing them out" in resistance
against the strangling pressure. I have been able
when making these tests to hang myself with a rope
and yet go on breathing for a considerable space of
time. This was due to the fact that my neck muscles
were so strong that I was able to "swell" them and
protect the wind-pipe frcm the rope's pressure.

Of course I do not wish to be understood as recom-
mending this severe test to any of my readers, but it
shows what can be done in the way of strengthening
the neck muscles. Such a test would be altogether
too strenuous for anyone who has not been developing
his neck muscles for a long time. And it would also
be highly hazardous for any investigator who did not
take the precaution of having friends at hand who

stood ready to extricate him from his plight in case anything went wrong.

But there is another test that will answer as well, and which is not as risky. When you feel certain that the muscles of your neck are reasonably strong, tie a sash in a single knot around your neck, having the knot at the front of the throat. Give the ends of the sash to two friends who stand on either side of you. At a signal let them begin to pull lightly in opposite directions, thus tightening the rope and subjecting you to a mild strangling. See if you can tense your neck muscles so that your breathing is not interfered with seriously. The pulling of your friends can be made more severe as you find your neck growing in power, and a signal—such as clapping your hands— will be sufficient to stop the strangling at any moment when you find the sash is being drawn too tightly.

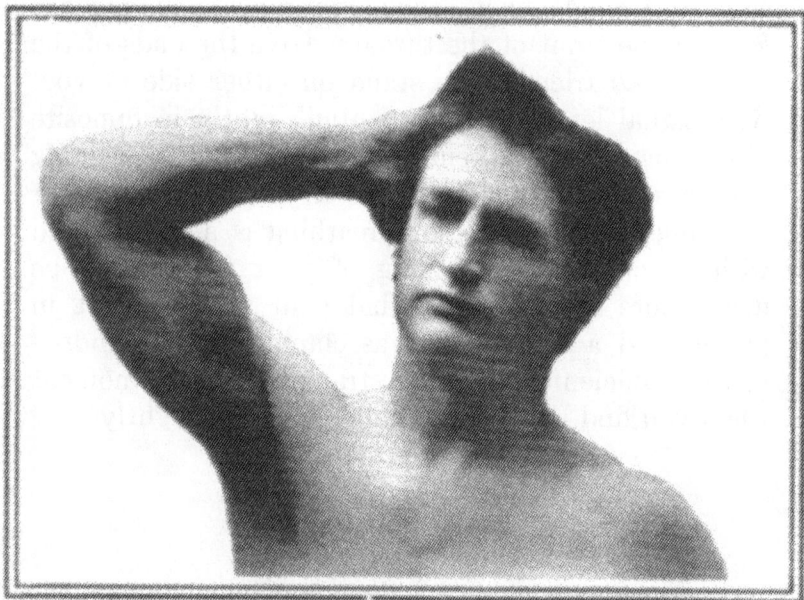

Photograph No. 44.

Exercise No. 24. Place the right hand on the right side of the head, as shown in the illustration. Now, resisting the movement slightly with the right arm, bring the head towards the right, (See next photo.)

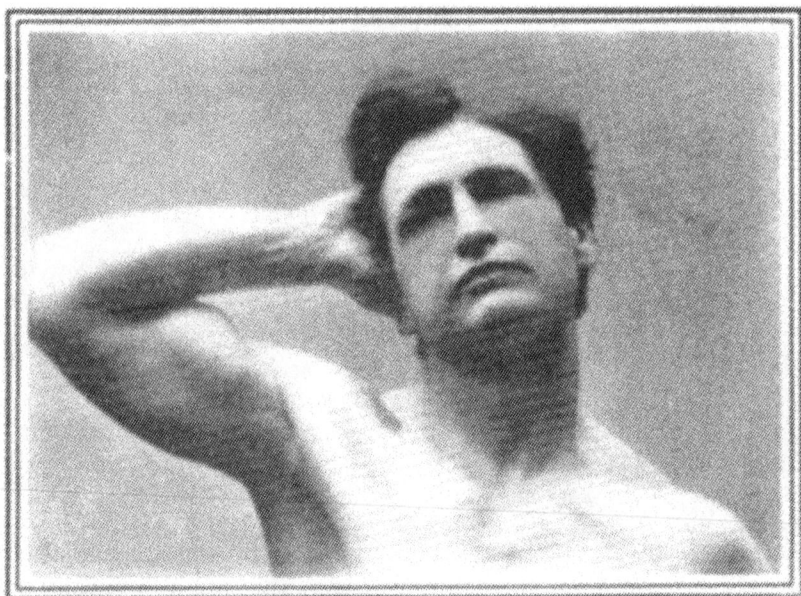

Photograph No. 45.

As shown in the above illustration. Take the same exercise with the left hand, pressing against the left side of the head. Continue each exercise until tired. This exercise develops the muscles on the sides of the neck.

This exercise can be taken slowly or speedily just as you may desire. If it is taken slowly and the muscles flexed very strongly, the development will appear more speedily.

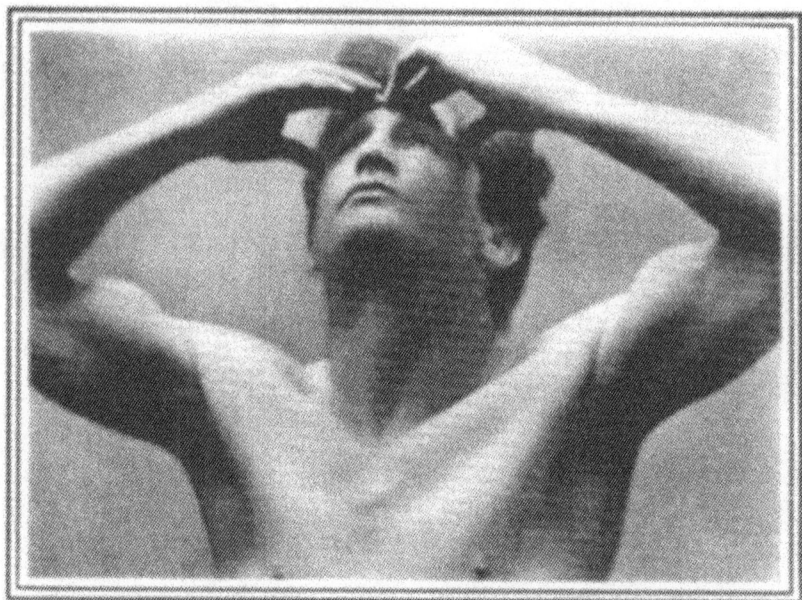

Photograph No. 46.

Exercise No. 25. Place the fingers of right and left hands on the forehead as shown in the above illustration. Be sure to start with the head as far back as possible. Now, resisting the movement slightly by pressing the fingers against the forehead, bring the head forward and downward. (See next photo.)

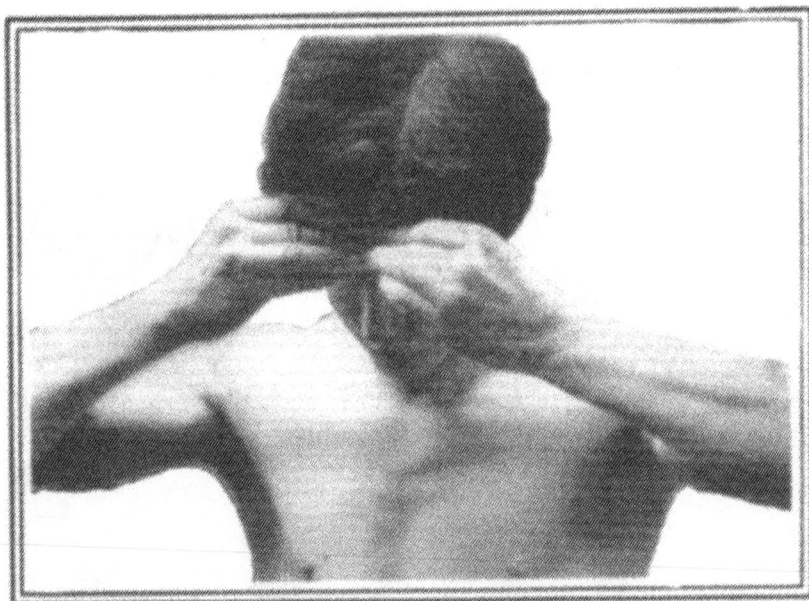

Photograph No. 47.

To the position shown in the above illustration. Continue the exercise until the muscles are slightly tired. This exercise is for developing the muscles on the front part of the neck.

This exercise can be varied slightly by bringing the head forward to the right, then bringing the head forward to the left. The movement can be taken slowly or fast as you may desire, though the remarks in the preceding movements apply also to this.

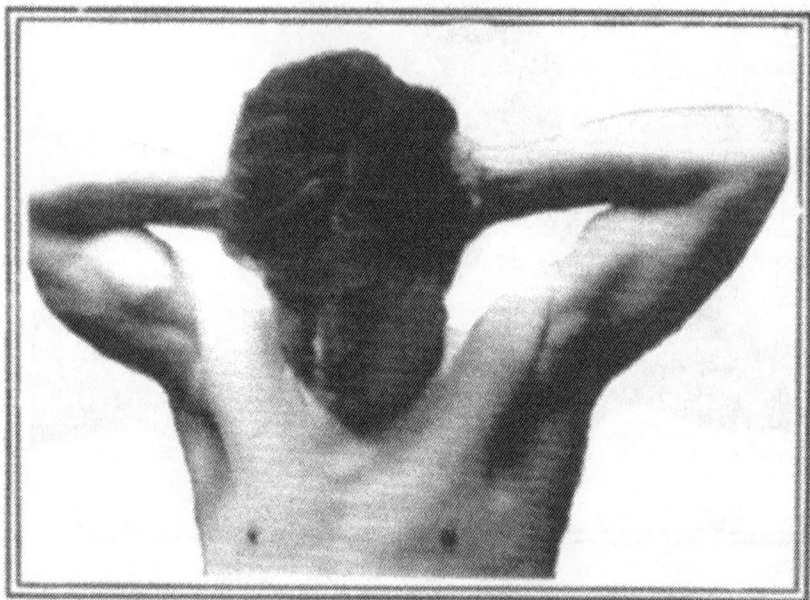

Photograph No. 48.

Exercise No. 26. Interlace the fingers behind the head and then bring head far forward until the chin almost touches the chest, as shown in above illustration. Now, resisting the movement slightly with the arms, press the head as far back as you can. (See next photo.)

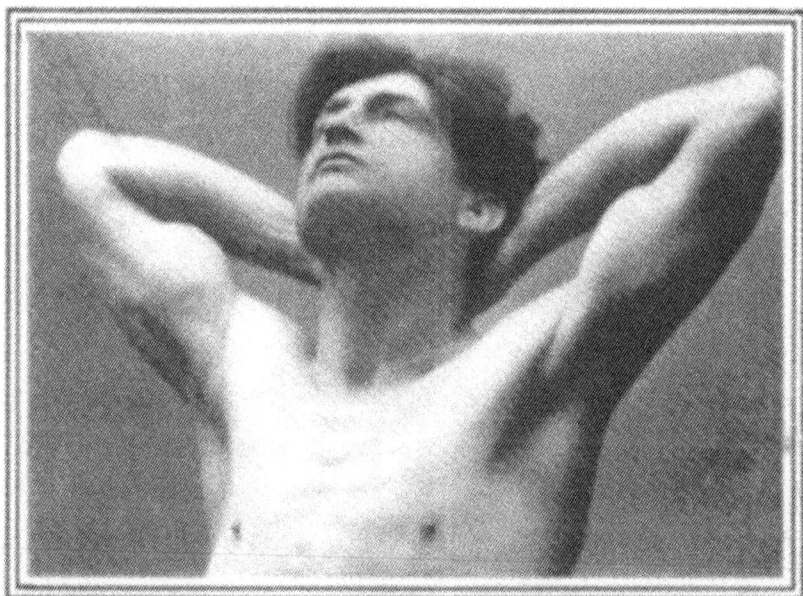

Photograph No. 49.

As shown in the above illustration. Continue the exercise until the muscles are slightly tired. This movement develops the broad muscles on the back part of the neck.

This exercise can be varied slightly by turning the head from the right to the left, while the above position is maintained. This movement is especially beneficial for strengthening the muscles that are used in wrestling. The muscles on the back of the neck must be very strong in order to resist the many difficult holds that are used in this strenuous exercise. To get the best possible results from the exercise be sure to bring the head far forward when the movement is made.

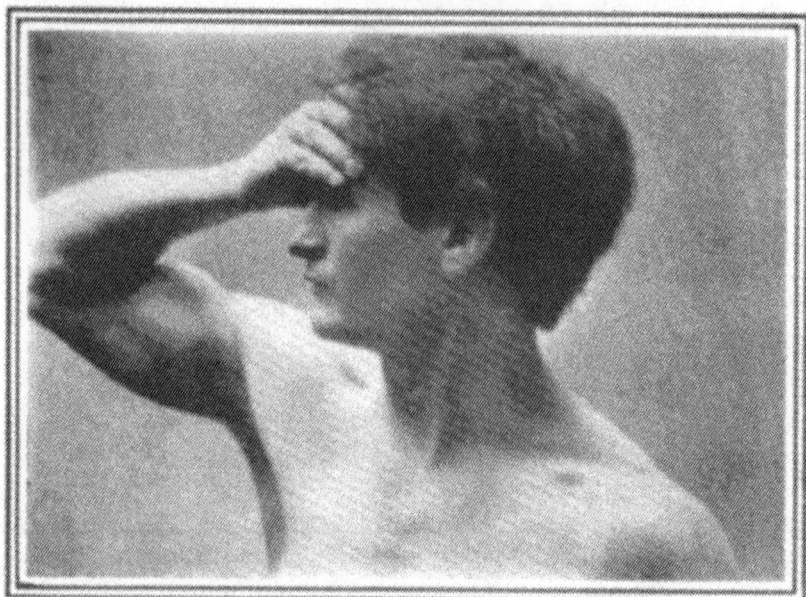

Photograph No. 50.

Exercise No. 27. With the head turned well to the right, press the fingers of the hand tightly around and against the forehead, as shown in the above illustration. Now, resisting the movement slightly with the arm, turn the head from the extreme right to the extreme left. (See next photo.)

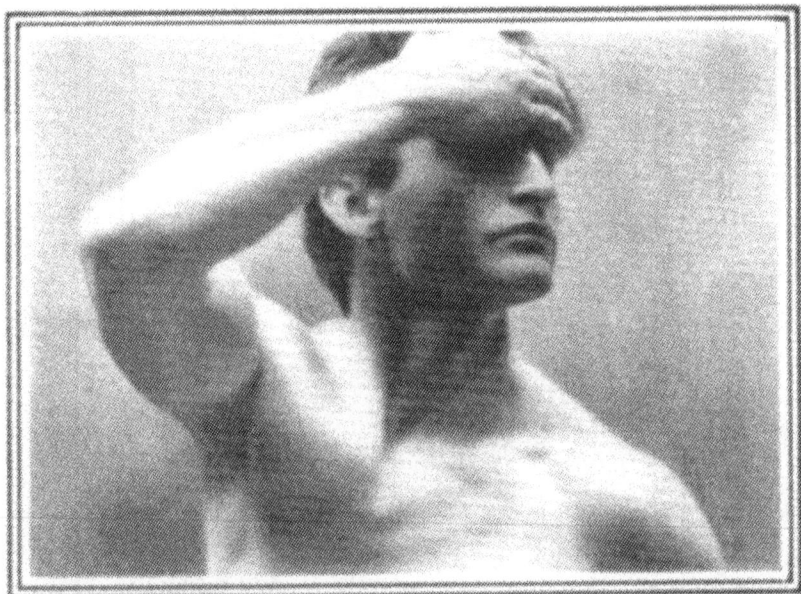

Photograph No. 51.

As shown in the above illustration. Take same exercise with positions reversed, using the left arm instead of the right. Continue each movement until the muscles are slightly fatiguec. This exercise develops the muscles that twist the head from side to side and which are located on both sides of the neck. The action of these muscles can be seen plainly during this move ment.

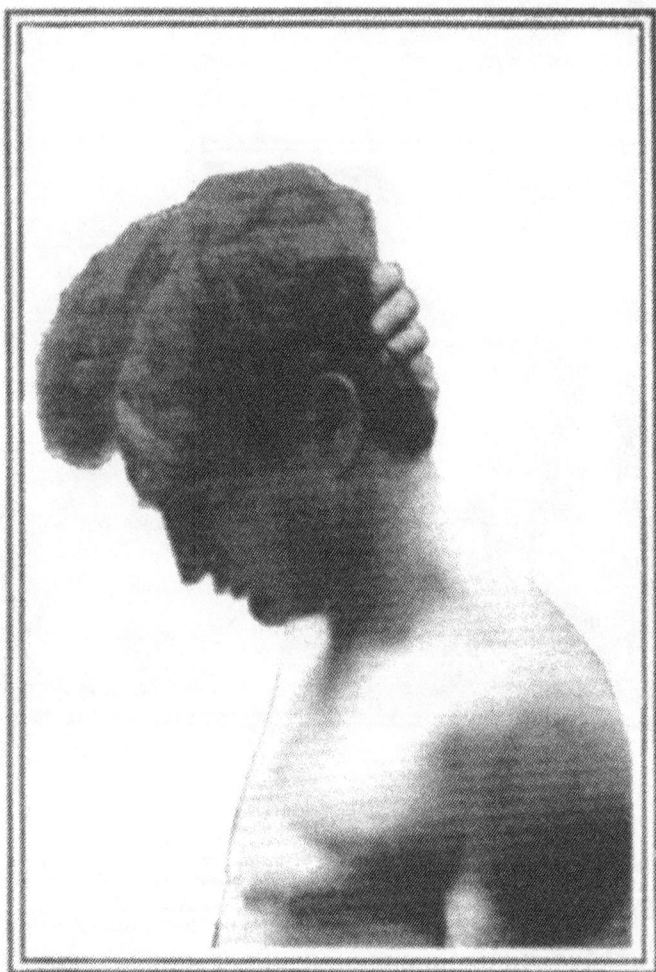

Photograph No. 52.

Exercise No. 28. With the head inclined far forward, place right hand as shown in above illustration. Now, pressing slightly against the movement, bring the head backward over towards the left shoulder, (See next photo.)

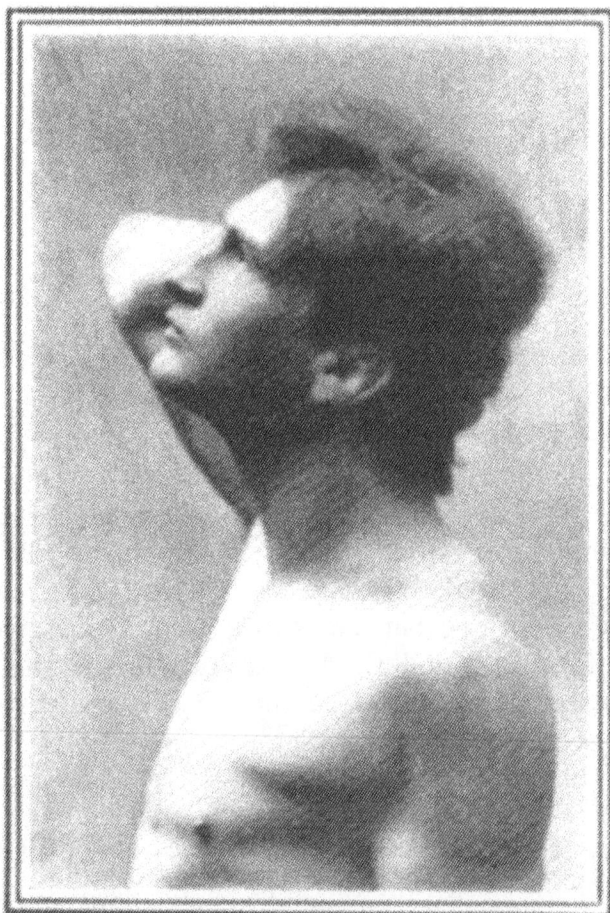

Photograph No. 53.

As shown herewith. Same movement, bringing head backward toward right shoulder, then forward and back again over left shoulder. Continue alternately from one side to the other until the muscles are tired. This exercise is for the broad muscles on the back of the neck and those converging with the slope of the shoulders. It can be varied by using the left hand instead of the right, or by using both hands, if desired.

This is another exercise that can be most emphatically recommended for those who are desirous of strengthening the muscles of the back of the neck that are used so vigorously in wrestling. In fact, these muscles should be well-developed if one desires a proper carriage and wishes the body to appear well-formed in every way. Very frequently the lack of development of these muscles makes one appear round-shouldered.

CHAPTER XVI.

Anatomical Structure of the Back Muscles.

As the very foundation of the structure of the back we have, of course, the spine or "back-bone." This is undoubtedly the most peculiar bony structure in the body. It is a "column" composed of twenty-four parts, each known as a vertebra. Seven of these vertebræ belong to the neck, and five to the lumbar region, or "small of the back." The other twelve, which are located between the cervical or neck vertebræ at the top and the lumbar vertebræ at the base of the spine, are known as the dorsal vertebræ—that is, they belong to the back proper.

Further, the bony encasement of the back is completed by the ribs, a pair of ribs running from each of the twelve dorsal vertebræ. It is over this framework of the back that the muscles are situated in five layers. There are thirty-two pairs of these back muscles in all, but most of these are of interest only to the surgical anatomist or other scientist, and I shall confine myself, in this chapter, to a discussion of those only that are of direct interest to the athlete.

While the splenius muscles are true back muscles, their influence is much felt in the muscular workings of the neck and for that reason I described them in Chapter XIV. The trapezius muscle, which I mentioned also in the same chapter, must now come in for a little closer attention. This is a broad, flat muscle, triangular in shape.   Its origin is in the back of the head, in the neck, and in all of the dorsal vertebræ— that is in all of the vertebræ of the back proper.   This will give an excellent idea of the great extent of this muscle, and a still further idea thereof may be gained from the fact that its insertion is in the collar bone and in the upper part of the shoulder blade.

Drawing the arms backward and downward is the main use of this muscle.   It also aids in the familiar act of shrugging the shoulders.   When the shoulder blades are drawn closer together it is the trapezius muscle that is employed.

The other great muscle of the back enjoys the rather formidable name of latissimus dorsi, but it is so important in the well developed back as to make it a great deal more worthy of admiration than its name suggests.

This muscle covers most of the back between the armpits and the hips.   It is splendidly developed in the habitual swimmer, for it is the muscle most used in keeping afloat in the water.   It is known also as the "climber's muscle," since it is greatly used in this form exertion.   It is a muscle that yields most readily to exercise and is capable of extraordinary development.

The origin of this muscle is extensive.   It arises from the six lower back vertebræ, from the lumbar vertebræ and from the crest of the hip bone.   There are also fleshy attachments to the three or four lower ribs.   From its various sources it becomes a perfect network of muscular fibres running in different directions.   The insertion, by means of a four-sided tendon that is some three inches in length, is in the humerus or upper bone of the arm.   Its workings may be felt in a back whose muscles are tensed, but it may be seen in action in the back of any athlete, though more particularly in that of the strong swimmer.

The rhomboid muscles are of interest to the athlete, since these are shown very prominently in the back of a man who is superbly developed. The rhomboids are capable of quick development, too. They are used in backward movements of the head and shoulders. They are seen to best advantage, perhaps, in the back of an athlete who is engaged in a stubborn, spirited tug-of-war.

If you wish to show the rhomboids as their best, let your upper arms hang at the sides, hold the forearms horizontally forward and clench the fists, tense your arm and back muscles, and force the elbows and shoulder blades firmly back. The tendons of the rhomboids will then show in parallel, perpendicular ridges between the shoulder-blades.

From the foregoing paragraph it may be inferred, with reason, that rowing is one of the ideal exercises for developing the rhomboids. All of the back muscles come in for a share of the benefit derived from the use of oars, but it is the rhomboids that are more particularly affected.

There are two muscles grouped under the general name of rhomboids. The uppermost is the rhomboid minor. It has its origin at the seventh of the neck vertebræ and the topmost dorsal vertebræ, while the insertion is at the spine of the shoulder blade. Immediately below is the major rhomboid, which has its origin from the four or five uppermost dorsal vertebræ while the insertion is at the shoulder blade.

Every one of the muscles that I have described in this chapter may be seen plainly through the skin when the muscular system of a well-developed back is being employed in vigorous work. Every one of these muscles plays a part in the natural work of the back—which is burden-bearing in one or another of its forms. In lifting, too, as in climbing, swimming, running, in tugging and hauling, or in resisting a tug, the strength of these muscles is the main factor in determining the victor. Wrestling provides every possible form of exercise for the muscles of the back.

It is highly proper to refer to the back as the seat, the center, of the whole muscular system, for the muscular strength of the entire trunk, and the effectiveness of all of the muscles in the arms and the legs depend upon the strength of the back. In, fact, the development of this portion of the body is absolutely essential to general physical strength.

It is in the back that weakness of the general muscular system is felt first when the strength is overtaxed, as in walking or by manual toil. It is the muscular system of the back, therefore, that should receive the first attention of the man who is trying to build up his muscular power.

At the outset of back-work, look for the development of the rhomboids. Nearly every man has some visible development of these. As the work goes on, look for more and more prominence of the muscles, and do not be satisfied unless you are able to easily note it.

Soon after beginning back work watch the gradual increase in size of the latissimus dorsi. Do not think of being satisfied unless the improvement of this muscle is decidedly noticeable. These two muscles, controlling as they do, most of the action of the back, *must* be *made* to thrive.

The improvement in the trapezius muscle is to be noted with interest, but it is certain that, when the latissimus dorsi and the rhomboids are brought to their best development, the trapezius will be found to have "looked after itself ' and to have shared in the general benefit.

CHAPTER XVII.

Exercises for Developing the Muscles of the Back.

In the photographs that belong to this chapter, those numbered from 54 to 60, is shown very clearly the system of work that is needed for the most effective development of the muscles of the back.

Take photograph 55 as a sample. This starts with the exact position of the most laborious burden bearing, and at the same time, with the hands in position for lifting. The next photograph shows the back enduring a strain consequent on the imaginary burden having been lifted.

In this exercise it is, of course, intended that the resistance given by the leg to the hands shall be increased gradually from day to day, the amount of such increase being best left to the judgment of the man in training. At all times, and in all forms of resistant muscle work, the resistance should be as great as may be overcome with comfort. For it follows that the greater the resistance, the more the benefit to the muscle employed in overcoming it—this always with the proviso that the resistance be not carried to the point of causing undue fatigue.

The next exercise, as shown by photographs numbered 57 and 58, is intended to bring the muscles of the back and various other parts of the body into full and hard play. The strain upon these muscles is a slow but continuous one that makes for great endurance. By continuing the exercise as long as may be done with comfort, quick development, especially of the climbing muscle, is assured. This should be made a favorite exercise by all of my readers who are anxious to acquire general muscular strength. It would be difficult to carry this exercise to a point where one would have too much of it, for the arm and leg muscles, the abdominal muscles, and, to some extent, those of the neck, shoulders and chest all come in for a share in development. Even the toes are considerably strengthened by frequent repetitions of this drill.

In photographs 59 and 60, illustrative of exercise thirty-two, the rhomboids, of which I have written, are seen just between the shoulder blades. In the first photograph they are shown somewhat, but in the second they are displayed with considerably more prominence. These muscles, which are so well worthy of development, are benefited very much by this particular exercise, giving them as it does, ideal work. If it is possible, perform this drill before a triple mirror so arranged that one of the folds will readily reflect the motions of the rhomboids. The mirror will also be of aid to you in noting their gradual development.

All of the back exercises should be performed energetically. Anatomically, the back is adapted admirably to vigorous work, and hence not very much work of the right kind conscientiously done, is needed to make the back begin to endure hard work without fatigue.

Whenever you are able to wind up a bout of exercise with a swim—and even in winter there are swimming pools available in our cities—remember that you are serving not only cleanliness but giving the back more exercise of an excellent kind.

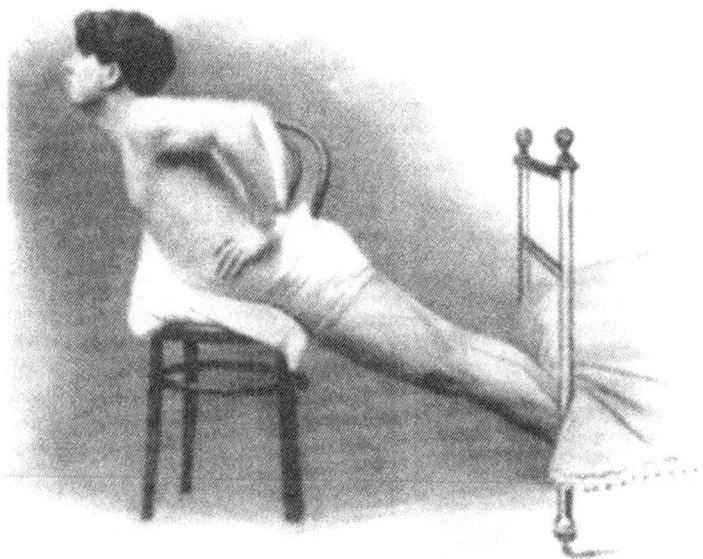

Photograph No. 54.

Exercise No. 29. Assume position as shown in illustration, putting the heels under the cross-pieces of the bed, hands on hips. Now, bend forward as far as you can, then raise as high as you can. Each time you raise upward, hold the body in this position a moment before returning. Continue the exercise until a feeling of fatigue in induced. In this exercise, if you place the chair far enough back, so that the weight of the body rests upon the thighs of the leg, the exercise will require much more effort. Also, when regaining the upward position, if you will stretch your arms far out in front, it will add to the difficulty of the exercise. Placing your hands on the back of the head while taking the exercise will also increase its difficulty.

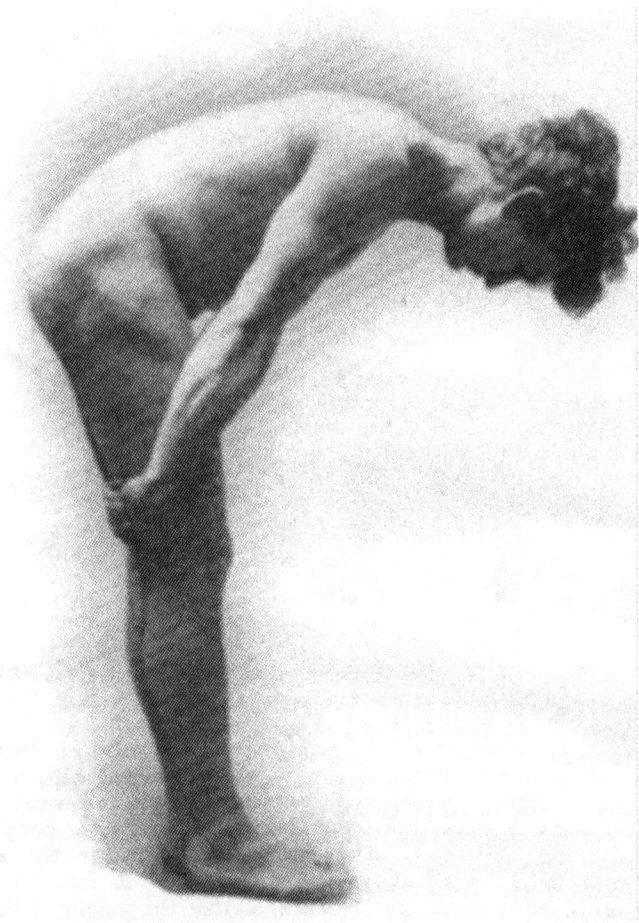

Photograph No. 55.

Exercise No. 30. Interlace the fingers under right leg as shown in illustration (See next photo.)

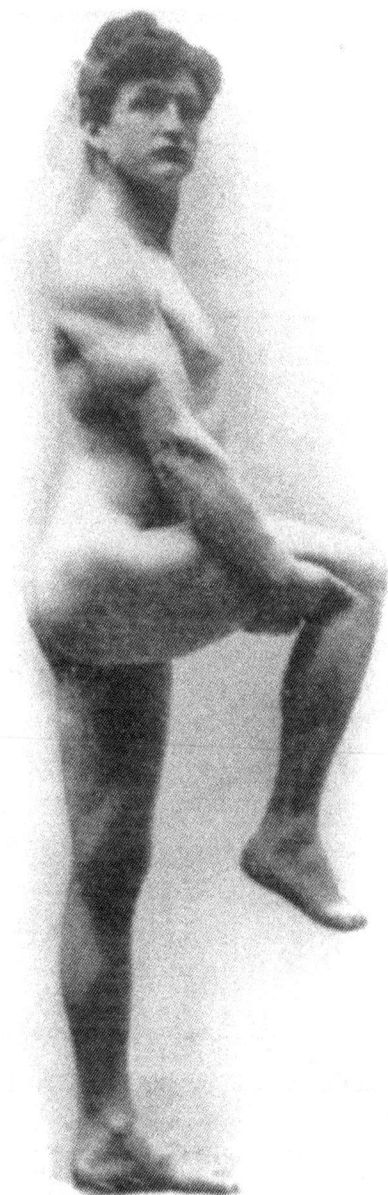

Photograph No. 56.

Then raise to position shown in above photo, slightly resisting
the movement with the leg. Make several movements shown in this
way, then interlace the fingers under the other leg and take similar
exercise. This exercise is particularly beneficial for strengthening the
muscles of the back about the waist line, ordinarily called the "small"
of the back.

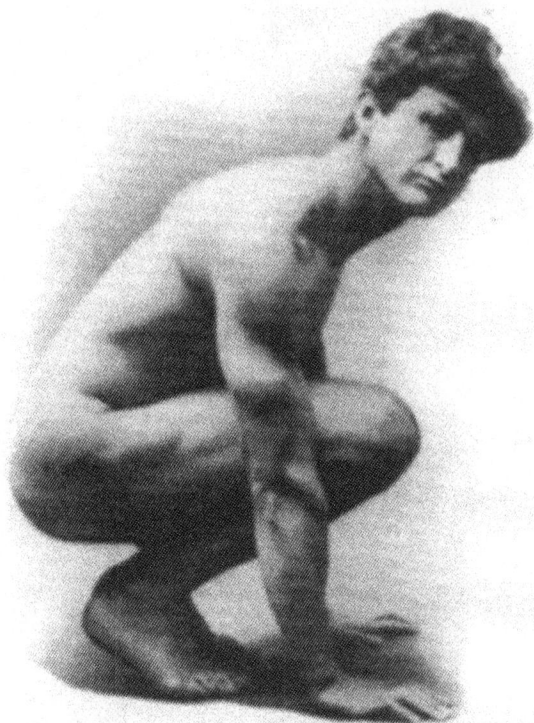

Photograph No. 57.

Exercise No. 31. From a standing position crouch as shown in photo, with hands placed on the floor. Now lean forward, bearing considerable weight on the hands, and then shoot the legs out (See next photo.)

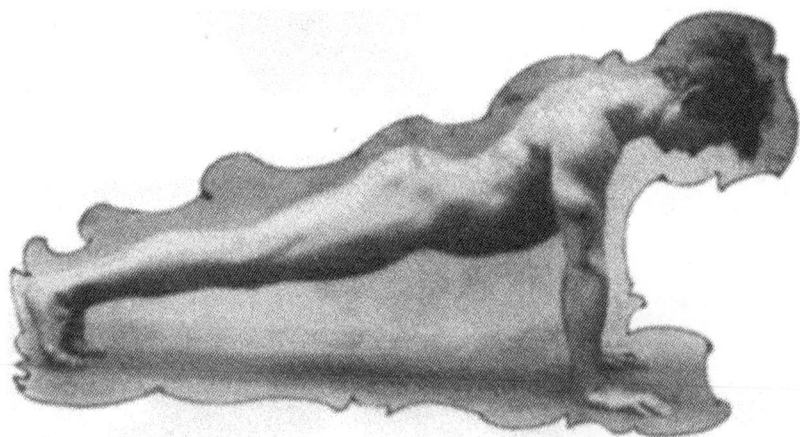

Photograph No. 58.

To the position shown in the above photo. Then return to starting position. Repeat until the muscles are quite fatigued.

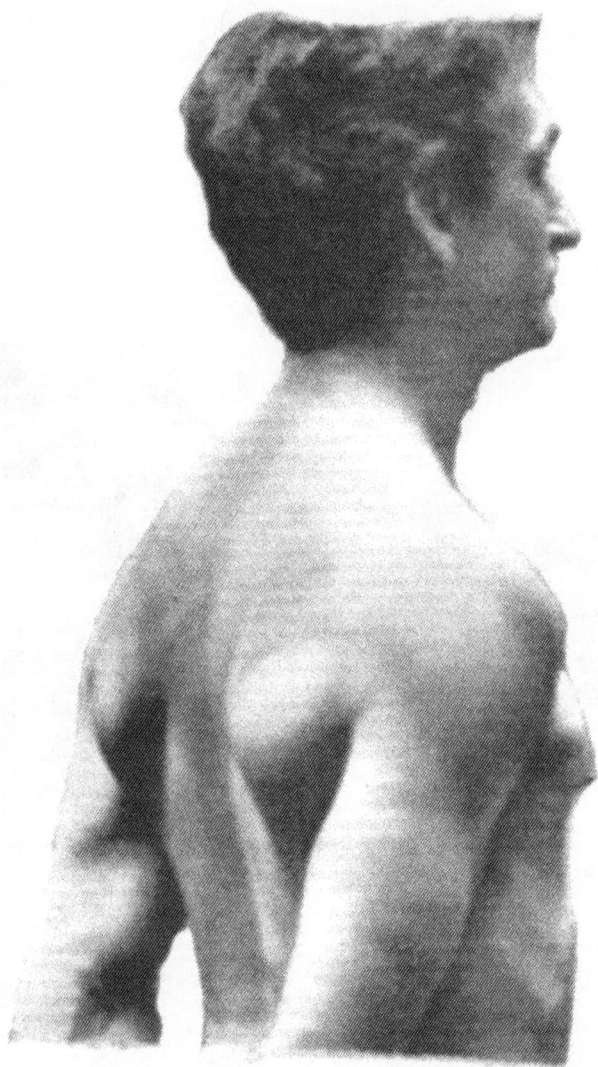

Photograph No. 59.

Exercise No. 32. Bring the shoulders as far forward and downward as you can, and also bring the head slightly forward. Now, with hands grasped together tightly, slowly bring the shoulders and the head backward as far as you can (See next photo)

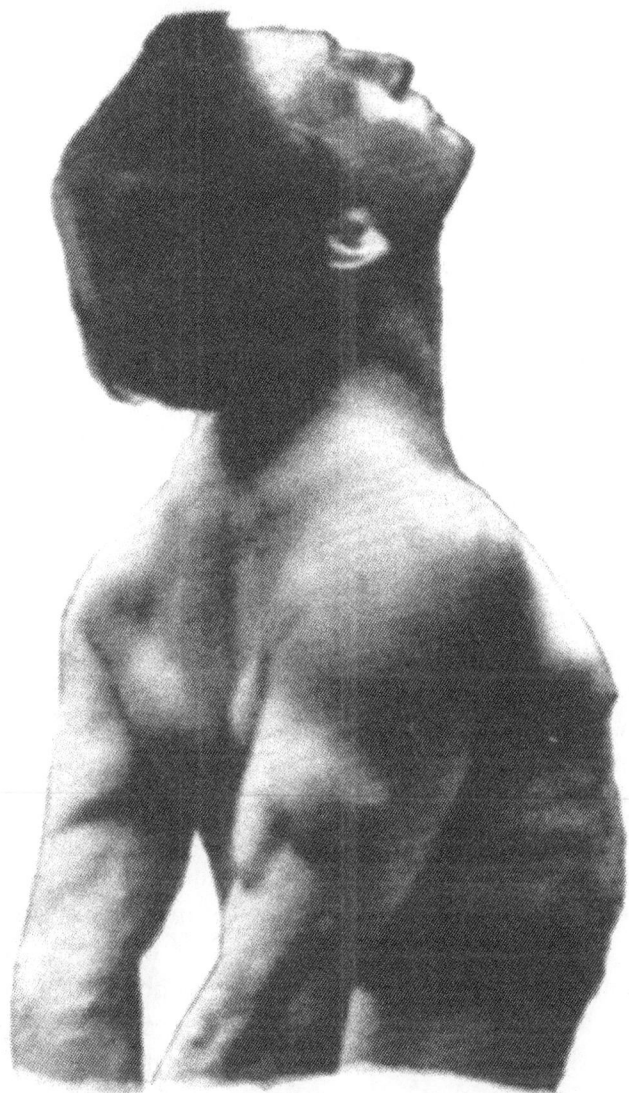

Photograph No. 60.

To the position shown herewith. Take this exercise slowly, and with the muscles strongly flexed. This is especially valuable for remedying round shoulders and will be found to affect very quickly the muscles that are used in maintaining a proper position of the shoulders. Continue the exercise each time until the muscles are thoroughly tired. Frequently when the shoulders are in a normal condition, they still have a round appearance if the muscles at the back of the neck are not developed. This exercise of the neck will be inclined to remedy this defect.

CHAPTER XVIII.

ANATOMICAL STRUCTURE OF THE ABDOMINAL MUSCLES.

At first thought it might seem to the student of physical training that if there were any muscles of the body that could be safely neglected, they would be those of the abdomen. Of what special use, if any, he may ask, are these same muscles?

The answer is that they are of tremendous importance in the total scheme of the system. In first place, they are a part of the general connective plan of the muscular body. Is is an axiom that any machine is only as strong as its weakest part, and to this truth the human body is no exception. In the act of deep breathing the abdominal muscles aid in throwing up that odd muscle, the diaphragm, and exercise of the former tends to strengthen the latter. Strength in the abdominal muscles makes the act of bending less fatiguing, too.

But most important of all the benefits that come from the exercise of the muscles in question, is that by which the involuntary muscles of the digestive system are affected for good.

How is it that the stomach and the small intestine accomplish their task of digesting the food that we eat? The mechanical portion of this work is accomplished by the action of the involuntary muscles that serve to keep the stomach and the small intestine in motion during the act of digestion. This mechanical action of the muscles named is necessary in order that the

148

food, in process of digestion, may be thoroughly mixed with the gastric and other digestive fluids. Such muscles act without any conscious effort of the will. Indeed, we are never conscious of their almost ceaseless workings.

Now, these involuntary muscles need exercise in order to keep them strong and healthy. The ordinary work that they do in digesting food is not sufficient. They must be helped in some other way. They must be made to work *through their neighbors, the voluntary muscles*. The instant that the voluntary muscles of the abdomen begin to contract and relax in exercise, the involuntary muscles near them are forced to perform the self-same work of contracting and relaxing.

Natural man, who lived an out-of-door life of hard toil and of the chase, did not need any especial exercise for the abdominal muscles. His daily life supplied all the exertion that was needed, and both the voluntary and the involuntary muscles of the abdomen were thereby strengthened.

But to-day, with most of us, conditions are vastly different. Our methods of living make it necessary for us to gain proper muscular development through devoting much of our leisure to special exercises, and to life out-of-doors. Hence it is needful that we pay serious attention to work that will give to our abdominal muscles the strength and endurance that must go with perfect health. Unless we do this we cannot hope for the needed conditions of vital strength and power.

Right here I wish to interpolate a word of warning. Many athletes—and even teachers, who should know better—indulge in the practice of taking a deep breath to bring the abdomen well in, and then walking or performing some other exercise while holding the abdomen well drawn in. Too much cannot be said against this practice. It is not only harmful, but is opposed to all common sense. Let the abdomen hang just as it naturally will during deep breathing and exercising, as at all other hours of the twenty-four. Holding in the abdomen unnaturally and forcibly can have but one effect—to compress the contents of the abdomen and to constrict the development of the intestines. *It is harmful to the last degree!*

Anatomically, the abdominal muscles may be said to consist of two layers, the superficial and the deep. As is the case in other portions of the body, the student of muscular development may content himself with a study of those muscles near the surface, those deeper in the flesh being governed in their improvement by the same kind of exercise that develops the superficial muscles.

The linea alba, or "white line" is the name given to a long and rather thin tendon that runs directly up the front of the abdomen from the crotch to the region of the chest muscles and which includes in its course, the region of the navel. It is placed between the two recti muscles, at either side of the front of the abdomen. Near the base of the abdomen the two recti muscles are close together and the linea alba is correspondingly narrow. As the recti ascend they become further apart, and the linea alba gets correspondingly wider.

On either side of the linea alba are the lineæ semi-lunares (half moon lines). These are just between the linea alba and either rectus muscle. The rectus abdominis is a long, flat muscle, extending along the whole of the front of the abdomen on either side of the linea alba. This muscle has attachment with the diaphragm, and is therefore used in the act of deep breathing.

All things considered, probably the external oblique muscle may be called the most important of the abdominal set. Tnis covers most of the side and fore part of the abdomen. It is a broad and thin muscle, and irregularly four-sided. The attachments of this muscle are numerous, and a description of all of the attachments would be bewildering to the novice in anatomy. But the statement that the muscle is attached to each of the eight lower ribs on either side will show why the act of deep breathing moves the abdomen so thoroughly. This muscle is known also as the descending oblique muscle, from the fact that its complicated origin is at the upper portions of the muscle.

Contrasted with this, is the internal oblique muscle, or the ascending oblique. The internal lies under the external, and is thinner and smaller, but of an irregular four-sided shape. This muscle, too, has a complicated origin and insertion, and it will be enough to state that part of the attachment is at the crest of the hip-bone. The purpose of this muscle is to draw the abdomen down again after it has been drawn up by the external oblique. The other two muscles of the superficial layer of the abdomen are the transversalis and the pyramidalis. They are of some importance in the muscular economy in that they aid the muscles already described, but they do not call for description in a work of the scope of this volume.

CHAPTER XIX.

Exercises for Developing the Muscles of the Abdomen.

Rational exercise for strengthening and developing the muscles of the abdomen must consist of feats that use those muscles with considerably more severity than is employed in the ordinary daily tasks of the would-be-athlete.

If one were to devise his own system of exercise, as I was compelled to do in order to obtain the best possible means of bodily development, it would be needful to study all of the varying movements that are demanded of the abdominal muscles in every day life. But in this work these muscular movements being separated and then classified, the system presented includes all of the movements in their proper order and rational proportion. The photographs that illustrate this chapter graphically show all the exercises required to bring about the best development of which the abdominal muscles are capable.

Exercise 33, as shown in photographs numbered 61 and 62, shows a form of work that is somewhat paralleled in gymnasiums by means of various ingenious and rather costly appliances. But as I have arranged the work, all the apparatus that is needed is found in any home—even in the hall bed-room of a lodging house.

This is a good sample of what the gymnastic instruc

tor means when he advises you to take more body work. You do not need to go to a gymnastic instructor for such advice, however, as the most perfect athlete is certain to be in need of such "body work." As many movements of this kind as can be taken without severe fatigue are advisable. The only caution to be given in connection with such work is the one that relates to the rush of blood to the head when the latter is held low. If there is such a rush, it shows that your development has not reached a satisfactory state and until such time, the bending should be performed with the head forward and chin resting on the chest.

More abdominal work is accomplished by following the preceding feat with exercise 34, which is explained by photograph 63. This hardens the abdominal muscles at the sides, particularly the external and internal obliques.

These two exercises furnish wholly satisfactory abdominal work. They should be kept up with great regularity and persistence, and may be depended upon to repay the student with most gratifying results. Not only do they add to the general scheme of muscular development; but they work out results in functional vitality that are soon perceptible, and which are little short of marvellous.

But there are sure to be those adventurous ones who will want "something harder." To such I offer exercise 35, which is depicted in photograph 64. A single trial will convince you that this is, indeed, "something harder." I do not recommend this exercise to every aspiring athlete. Many will find it altogether too severe at first. In that case it will be safer to content yourself for quite a long time with the preceding exercise, reserving number 35 until the general strength of the body makes it possible to take it up without injury to yourself.

Bear in mind, throughout your training, that any exercise, which results in decided straining is bound to be harmful. Those who have made a careful study of physical development realize to the full, the difference between "training" and "(s)training."

Of course the enthusiast who strains at his exercise is perhaps only trying to hurry his development. He thinks that by thus exerting himself to the extreme limit of his powers he will force the growth of muscular tissue that much faster. And it is true that one can to an extent force the rapid building of muscle by unusually strenuous efforts. But this can be done by systematic and persistent work, and for the enthusiast to carry his exercises so far as to strain himself, or reach his very limit of strength, is not only unnecessary but positively injurious. Tremendous strength cannot be built up in a day or a week, or even a month. It is an utter impossibility. If ever achieved it will come as a slow growth. It will take months and years of faithful training to finally arrive at the summit of one's powers, and as soon as you thoroughly realize this truth you will settle down to steady, persistent, but at the same time, energetic work, free from all violent and spasmodic efforts.

And while it is certainly true that it requires the vigorous use of the muscles to develop them, yet overwork at any time will only exhaust one's energies. It will tear down the muscles faster than they can be built up, faster than one can recuperate. The result will be that you simply will wear out. It is against this that the enthusiastic beginner must guard himself. He has only a definite amount of vitality to depend upon.   And when he has found by experience just the amount of strenuous exercise which he can stand, without exerting himself too much, he will then be in a position to build the very best of health, and a perfect and beautiful physique.

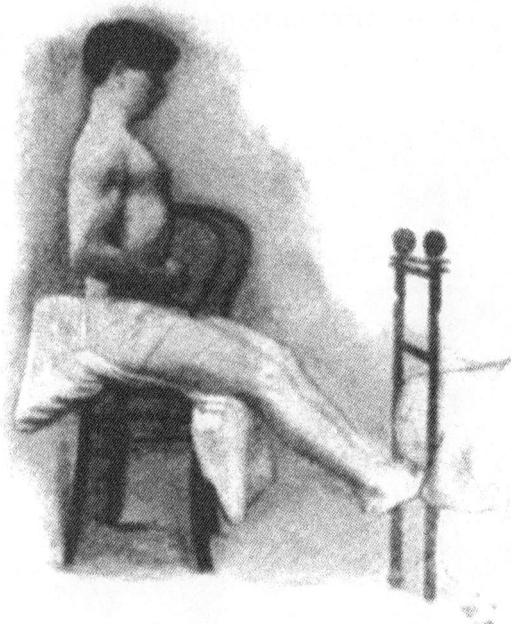

Photograph No. 61.

Exercise No. 33. After securing a chair, on which a pillow
or cushion should be placed, put your feet under the cross-
pieces of the bed, clasping your hands together over abdomen
as shown in illustration. Now bend backward (See next photo)

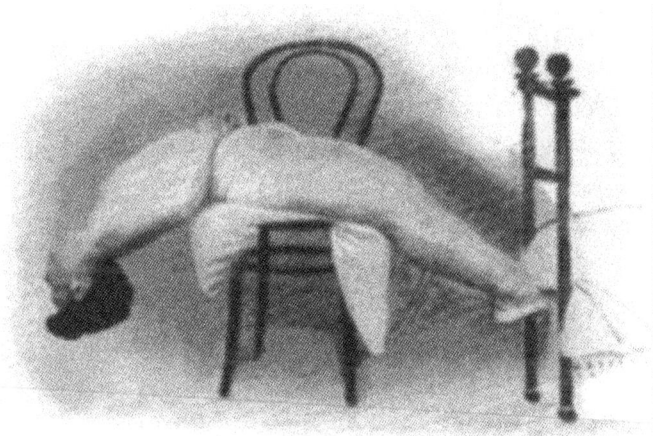

Photograph No. 62.

to the position shown in the above illustration. Rise to
the former position, and continue the exercise until tired. If
the exercise makes you dizzy when holding your head back in
this manner, keep your head forward, your chin on your chest,
during the entire movement.

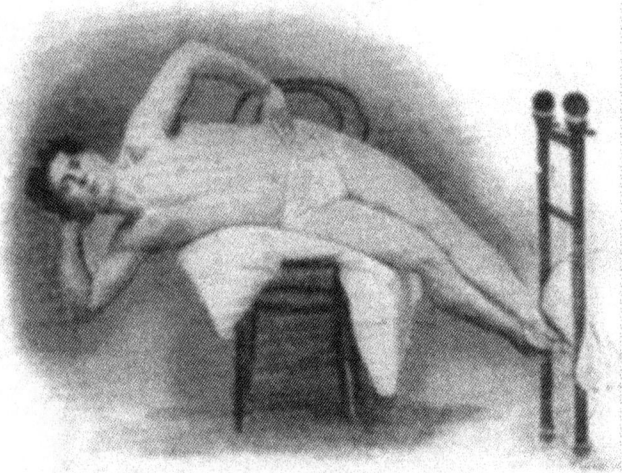

Photograph No. 63.

Exercise No. 34. Recline on your right side, crossing your left leg over the right, and placing both feet under the cross-pieces of the bed, as shown in illustration. Now, bend down as far as you can, then rise as nearly as you can to a sitting position, keeping your body in a sidewise position during the entire movement. Continue until a feeling of fatigue is induced. Same exercise with the position reversed, reclining on the left side.

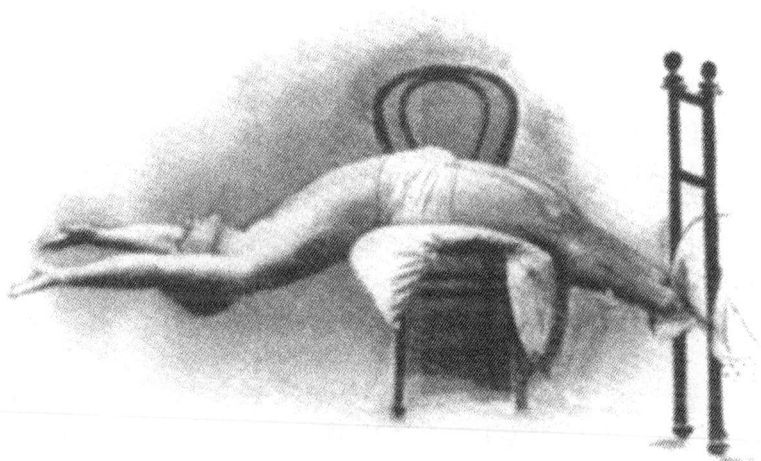

Photograph No. 64.

Exercise No. 35. This is an exercise similar to No. 33, except that the arms should be stretched far outward, as shown in the illustration. Keep the arms in this position during the entire movement. I would not advise anyone, unless very strong, to attempt this exercise.

CHAPTER XX.

ANATOMICAL STRUCTURE OF THE HIP MUSCLES.

I venture to say that many who exercise daily, have been in the habit of regarding the hips as a region of the body which is of minor importance. Or else they console themselves with the reflection that "general bodily development will bring their share of work to the hips."

If you belong to the class of those who have worked for swelling biceps and sturdy legs, and have left the hips to take care of themselves, it is certainly high time that you came to your athletic senses. If one is to possess an all-around perfect body, the hips must have their own especial treatment and a lot of it at that.

Of what use are the hips? Well, in the first place, if it were not for the muscles of the hips you would not be able to maintain an erect position. In the next place, in striking or in hauling or lifting, a portion of the muscular force needed is derived from the muscles of the legs and hips. There is not an important movement of the body involving the general muscular system, wherein the hip muscles do not play a prominent part in the force with which the movement is made.

Remember this! In boxing, walking or running, riding, rowing, bicycling, in jumping or kicking, or in any athletic sports or pastimes, hip muscles must be developed if the best possibilities of power are desired.

160

In every arduous kind of manual labor, strong hip muscles are also demanded.

With the ancients, the hips were justly regarded as the seat of bodily power. A man gloried in his strong hips; they symbolized his manliness. Jewish warriors boasted that they had smitten their enemies hip and thigh—meaning thereby that they had utterly destroyed those who had opposed them. Strong hips have been always taken as denoting the possibilities of satisfactory reproduction of the human species. A man with powerful hips is likely to become the father of strong, vigorous children. A woman with well-developed hips is regarded as being far better fitted for the task of bearing healthy children than is a woman with narrow and weakly developed hips.

Perfect hips are accepted as one of the outward signs of perfect health, and well may this be so, for with such hips are generally found associated, organs that have been trained to meet the demands of life, and this is more especially true of the organs of digestion.

Let it be stated as an uncontrovertible truth that *the man or woman who has attained perfection of hip development is admirably fitted for the performance of every normal function of life!*

The osseous structure of the hips is composed of the two bones, one on either side of the body, and of the sacrum, that small, triangular bone that is wedged in between the hip bones at the back. These three bones form what is known as the pelvis, or basin of the trunk. Our lower organs are protected at the sides and back by this bony framework.

Of the muscles that belong distinctively to the hips there are nine on each hip. These are known as the gluteal muscles. In general, and in addition to the work of keeping the body in an erect position, the task of these muscles is to adduct or draw forward and extend the thigh, also to provide for the rotating movements of which the leg is capable.

I do not purpose describing all of the nine muscles to be found in this region. A knowledge of three of them will suffice for the athlete in training.

Stand with the back of one heel upon a table. Have the trunk of the body as far from the table as possible. Now, keeping the heel in the same position, raise and lower the pelvis alternately. With your fingers feel the play of the muscles over the buttocks. Then, in the same way, and with the same exercise, feel the play of the muscles at the side of the hips.

Now, standing on one leg, and with the foot of the other leg well clear of the floor, make this second leg move in all the rotating ways of which it is capable. While doing so, let your fingers glide over the hip muscles, noting the full play of all the muscles.

These experiments will give you a very good idea of what an important part the hip muscles play in the work of the body. If you have the opportunity, it will be an excellent idea to study with the finger tips the work of the same muscles in the hips of a man whom you know to be a good all-around athlete.

The first of the muscles that I am going to describe is known to anatomists as the gluteus maximus. (I dislike to make such frequent use of Latin names, but so far, the only names for most of the muscles in the body are the Latin ones that the anatomists have forced upon us. One of these days a physical culturist will devise a simpler set of names!) In a general way it may be said that this muscle is the one nearest the surface, and that it covers nearly all of the buttocks. It is an unusually broad muscle, and it is very thick and fleshy.

In shape this muscle is four-sided. The better it is developed the more prominent and firm the buttocks will be. For if the buttocks consist mostly of fat, and with very little evidence of muscle, it is an evidence of physical degeneracy with which no one should rest content.

This muscle is of very coarse structure, as it needs to be for the work that is assigned to it. It is made up of bundles of fibres that lie parallel to each other, and these are collected together in large bundles, so that the general formation might be said to be very much like bundles of twigs. All who remember the old fable of the strength that lay in a bundle of twigs as compared with the strength of a single twig, will understand what possibilities there are in the way of the development of this gluteus maxiums muscle.

The origin of this muscle is of so complex a nature as to be bewildering to one who cannot go deeply into the matter. In a general way it may be said that the muscle arises from the upper edge of the hip bone, from the sacrum—that little triangular bone that is wedged in between the two hip bones—and from the coccyx—the bony end of the spine. The origin is also from the muscle that serves to keep the spine erect. Some of its origin is also in ligaments and tendons of this region, and from some of the sheathings of other muscles.

The fibres of this great muscle run downward and outward to its insertion, which is also of a complicated nature. The general effect of this insertion, however, is to bind the thigh more thoroughly to the hip.

Of course, a muscle that is so much in use is subjected to a great deal of friction. This is met by the provision of three synovial bursæ, or sacks, which liberate such quantities of synovial, or lubricating, fluid as is needed to relieve the friction. One of these sacks is of considerable size, while the other two are smaller—one of them, indeed, being sometimes entirely wanting.

Second in importance to these hip muscles is the gluteus medius. This is a broad, rather thick and much radiated muscle that is situated along the outer surface of the upper portion of the hip bone, and just below the crest of that bone.

This muscle has its origin on the hip bone between the upper and the middle curved lines. From this origin, the fibres of the muscle gradually converge into a strong, flat tendon which is inserted in the upper portion of the thigh bone.

The first purpose that the gluteus medius muscle serves is the rotating of the leg. It also abducts the thighs; that is, spreads them further apart when they have been close together. Most important of all purposes in the way of general movement is that of making the thigh move forward, without which act walking and running would be impossible.

Smallest of all of the three muscles is the gluteus minimus. This is found immediately beneath the medius. It is shaped like a fan, and has its origin near the middle of the upper portion of the hip bone. The fibres converge to a deep tendon—the handle of the fan, so to speak—and this tendon is situated in the thigh bone. A single synovial sack furnishes the lubricating liquid for this muscle. The purposes of this muscle are to help the gluteus medius in the work that the latter does.

Thus, in the main, the movements of the hips and thighs have been accounted for in the muscles that I have described. It will be understood then, that the development of the hip muscles is very far from being unimportant for him who would possess the fullest degree of bodily strength and activity.

Naturally the reader will want to know how he can best learn whether his hip muscles are developed as well as they should be. Such tests can go hand in hand with the exercises that will be described in the next chapter. In other words, the exercises themselves will furnish the best guide. If these exercises induce fatigue easily, the hip muscles are in poor condition. The gradually acquired ability to endure more and more of this hip work will attest to the development of muscular power in this region.

CHAPTER XXI.

EXERCISES FOR DEVELOPING THE MUSCLES OF THE HIPS.

Now, here is an abundance of good, strong, health-giving and muscle-toughening work for the hips. Undoubtedly this work will cause a good deal of fatigue at first, and if it does you will have the sorry satisfaction of knowing that you have heretofore neglected a very important lot of muscles.

Keep at this work until no reasonable amount of it will fatigue you unduly. When you have reached that happy point in your physical development, still keep on in order to make sure that you will never again find your hip muscles away below par.

Start right in with exercise 36, which is depicted clearly in photographs 65 and 66. Here you are giving immediate employment to our friends of the last chapter, the gluteus medius and the gluteus minimus. Study the pictures quite a little while and then get down to the good, hard work of trying the exercises. Take my word for it, that, unless your hip muscles are in good condition, you will soon have a feeling of soreness that will clearly indicate to you just where the gluteus medius and minimus are located. When you have made a study of the illustrations and have practiced *thinkingly* at the exercise, you will understand fully why the work must benefit these two important muscles. I have used the word "thinkingly" with a purpose. I wish I could impress upon all of my readers the vast importance of always thinking when exercising. If you merely go through the work like an automaton you certainly throw away half of the benefit that is to be derived from it.

Think all the time! First study the illustrations and practice the exercises. That is learning the *how*. Be fully sure that you understand the *how*. Don't acquire a wrong method in doing a single one of the exercises. And, just as soon as you have mastered the *how*, set about learning the *why*. In other words, understand the *reason* for the exercise; demonstrate to yourself just how the exercise accomplishes the improvement in muscle that you desire. Understanding the *why* of a feat renders you incapable of going very far wrong in the matter of method.

Next glance at photographs 67 and 68, which illustrate exercise 37. Understand what is required of you, and see if you can figure out for yourself just what hip muscles are benefited by following the directions given.

If you can't figure it out, I will explain to you that the gluteus medius and minimus muscles are benefited very much in this work, and the gluteus maximus comes in for its share of the work also. If you do not realize this fully after trying the work, place your hand on the buttocks of a friend who is doing the same exercise, and you will see how the gluteus maximus is brought thoroughly into play. It will also be noted that the abdominal muscles are vigorously used in this exercise.

With the hints that I have already given it ought not to be difficult for you to understand the muscular improvement that must result from frequent use of exercise 38, shown in photographs 69 and 70.

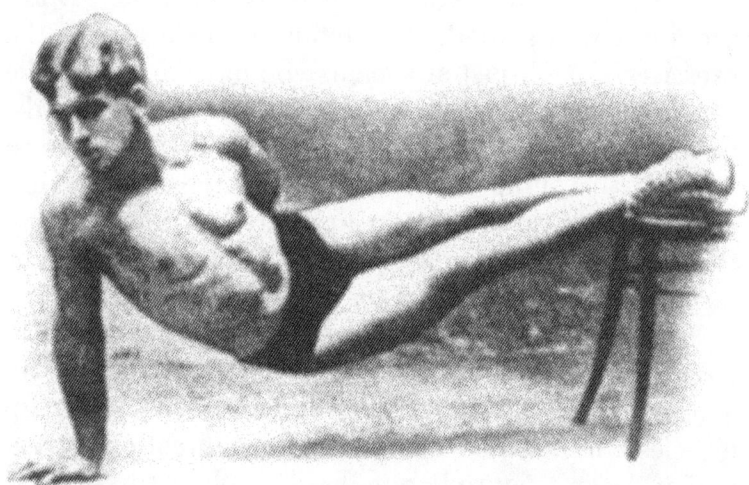

Photograph No. 65.

Exercise No. 36. With feet placed on chair or bed, rest body as in above position then rise as shown in next photograph.

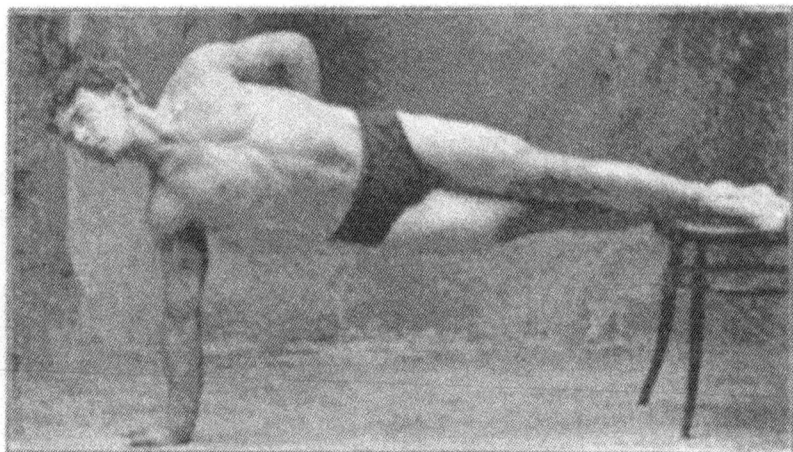

Photograph No. 66.

Continue until tired, then same exercise with weight resting on left arm.

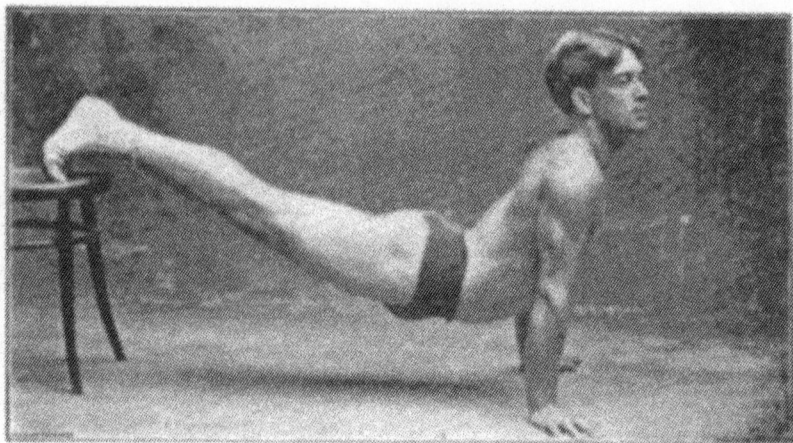

Photograph No. 67.

Exercise No. 37. Place feet on bed or chair, body resting
as above, then raise body as high as possible as shown in next
photo.

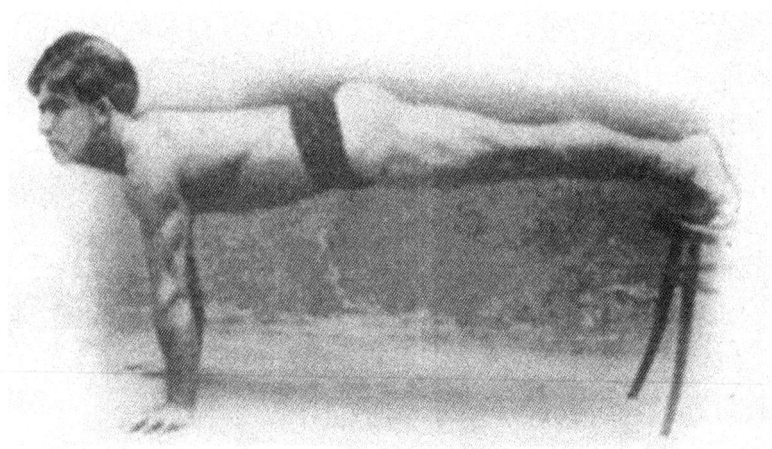

Photograph No. 68.

Repeat until the muscles are reasonably tired.

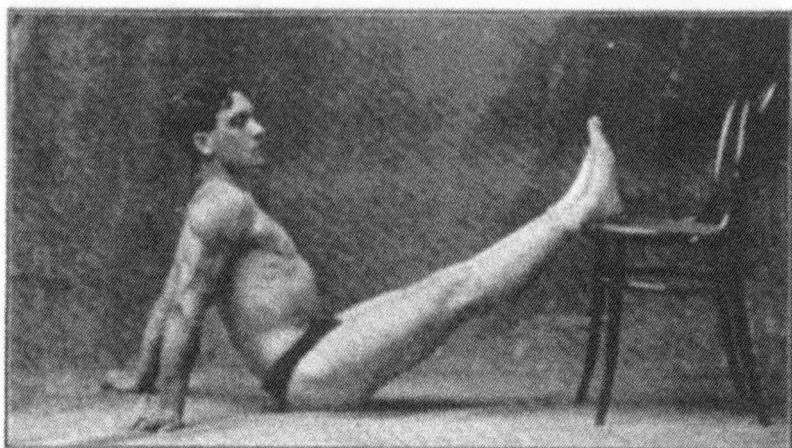

Photograph No. 69.

Exercise No. 38. With heels resting on chair or bed as above, raise body as high as possible, as shown in next photo.

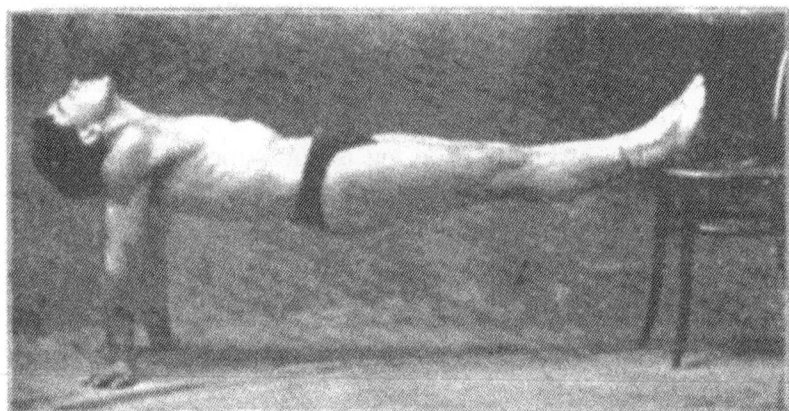

Photograph No. 70.

Repeat until muscles are tired.

CHAPTER XXII.

Anatomical Structure of the Upper Leg Muscles.

The upper leg extends from the hip to the knee. The basis of the upper leg is the femur, or thigh bone. The actions of this bone are controlled by some of the most powerful muscles in the body.

Near the surface of the leg is the superficial or outside fascia. As has been explained several times in this volume, a fascia is a membrane that forms a sheathing for muscles. This superficial fascia covers the upper leg; it is just beneath the skin, and consists of two layers, between which are found the surface blood vessels and nerves.

Clear away these two layers, and we come to the deep fascia, which, on account of its great extent, anatomists have termed the fascia lata. It covers the whole of the upper leg, and it usually varies in thickness according to the part of the limb where it is found.

Between the layers of this fascia lata is the first muscle of the upper leg to which I shall call your attention. This muscle is known as the tensor fasciæ femoris. It is found at the side of the leg, and its origin is at the crest of the hip bone on the outer side. About one-fourth of the way down the thigh bone the muscular tissue is inserted between two layers of the deep fascia mentioned above, and from this point the muscle is continued as a thick band of tendon that is

174

fastened, at last, to the tibia, or smaller bone of the lower leg.

Next we will consider the sartorius, or "tailor's muscle." It has received its nickname from the fact that it is the muscle much used by tailors when sitting cross-legged. This sartorius is the longest muscle in the body. It is flat and narrow—very much like a ribbon. When the leg is tensed, this muscle can be found running from the outside of the leg, beginning at the hip. It runs slantingly across the front of the leg, and considerably above the knee, then reaches the inner side of the leg and runs down to the knee.

This muscle has its origin in tendinous fibres. Near the point of insertion the broad tendon comes to the front of the knee, and the point of insertion is near the top of the tibia, or larger bone of the lower leg. The sartorius is one of the muscles that comes in for a very full share of work in all exercises or other movements that involve rising or squatting. The muscle is often extraordinarily developed in tailors.

There is just one more muscle to be considered in connection with the front of the upper leg, but it is of such importance that its consideration will take up considerable space. This is the quadriceps extensor muscle, which covers pretty nearly all of the front of the upper leg. It is a four headed muscle—that is, it has four points of origin—and its function is to extend (straighten) the leg. It would really be a group of four separate muscles, were it not that all of the portions unite below in a single tendon for insertion. The four parts of this muscle are known as the vastus externus, vastus internus, rectus femoris and the crureus.

The rectus femoris is found in the middle of the front of the leg. It arises from two heads, both on the hip bone. The vastus externus is the largest part of the quadriceps extensor. Its origin is in a network of fibres attached to the upper portion of the thigh bone and to the hip bone. The general course of the mus- is along the outer side of the leg and beneath the tendon of the tensor fasciæ femoris.

So close together are the vastus internus and the crureus that, on a careless examination, they appear to be one muscle; but dissection shows them to be separate. Their general course is along the front of the inner side of the leg.

The fibres of the vastus internus are directed down- ward. The crureus muscle has its origin at the front of the shaft of the thigh bone. As has already been stated, all four portions of the quadriceps extensor converge into a single tendon. This goes to the knee, and is attached to the knee cap.

At first thought it may strike my reader as somewhat strange to have the extensor muscles of the leg in the front, while in the upper arm the extensor muscle (the triceps) is at the back of the limb. The reason for this, however, will be understood by flexing first the arm and then the leg. In the case of the arm, the hand or fist is brought up in front of the body by the act of flexing. In flexing the leg, however, the heel is brought up toward the back.

In the hand, too, by way of contrast, the palm of the hand is uppermost in most actions, while, with the foot, the sole represents the palmar surface. Yet the bottom of the foot is not as pliable as is the hand. While the fingers can be folded over on the base of the hand, the sole (or palm) of the foot is not very flexible, and the toes can go but a little way toward the heel.

These things are thus on account of the different

work performed by the hand and the foot. The hand must be capable of adapting itself to a great variety of movements, while the work of the foot is confined practically to walking and running or to some modification of these tasks. In the same way the arm is capable of a far greater variety of movements than are possible to the leg. The general bony structures of an arm and a leg are so similar that we must look to evolution for an explanation of the difference in the number and extent of movements possible. In the ape, the foot is more like the hand; in the monkey, the similarity is even more marked. We can only understand that the slowly graded difference between the forms of muscular activity in man and in the ape have through centuries of usage, brought about the strongly marked differences between the arm and leg as we find them in man.

Below man, all of the animals, the ape included, use the upper limbs to a greater or less extent in the act of locomotion. In man, the legs only are used for locomotion, while the hands are employed solely in doing the finer executive work of the brain.

Thus, as the leg is used only for locomotion, we find the biceps of the upper leg at the rear instead of at the front as in the case of the arm.

The muscles of the back of the upper leg are called, collectively, the "hamstrings." As divided by anatomists, these muscles are classed as the biceps, the semitendinosus and the semimembranosus.

The biceps femoris, (biceps muscle of the thigh) as it is called by anatomists, is a large and long muscle. Its situation on the upper leg is at the back of the leg for the greater part of its course, but towards the knee it goes out toward the outer side of the limb. Its fibres can be felt plainly under the skin. One head of the muscle has its origin on the inner side of the hip bone and near its lower edge. The second and shorter head of this muscle arises from the thigh bone itself. The fibres of the longer head form a long "belly," which passes downward and ever so slightly outward toward the outer side of the leg. The two portions of the muscle join and are merged into a thick tendon that is inserted at the outer side of the head of the fibula, the small and outer bone of the leg. This tendon forms the outermost of the hamstrings.

The semitendinosus muscle is short in its fleshy part, and is to be observed for the great length of its tendon, which may be felt at the back and inner side of the upper leg. It arises from the hip through the same tendon that attaches the long head of the biceps. A little more than half way down the upper leg, this muscle passes into a long and round tendon which is inserted near the top of the tibia, or principal bone of the lower leg. This tendon is found behind the sartorius tendon.

Last of the hamstring muscles is the semimembranosus, which derives its name from the fact that the tendon of origin is somewhat of the character of a membrane. This tendon is thick, and arises from the lower portion of the hip bone. It is inserted near the head of the shaft of the tibia.

All of the hamstring muscles are employed in flexing the leg upon the thigh; hence their importance in locomotion is fully as great as that of the quadriceps extensor muscle at the front of the leg. When the knee is only half flexed the action of the biceps is to rotate the leg slightly outward—a familiar movement in walking or running. On the other hand, the semitendinosus, and to some extent the semimembranosus muscle, work to rocate the leg inward.   The hamstrings can therefore be studied best with the fingers when rotating the leg.

These muscles also help to keep the pelvis properly in place on the thigh bone.   At the same time they draw the trunk backward.   This can be noted when rising from a stooping position.   The effect is observable to an exaggerated degree when the trunk is bent so far over backward as to form an arch of the body.

CHAPTER XXIII.

EXERCISES FOR DEVELOPING THE MUSCLES OF THE UPPER LEGS.

Leg exercises may be had in the greatest variety. I present seventeen photographs illustrating the movements in the exercises which, after long experience, I have found to be the best of all for developing to practical perfection the muscles of the upper leg.

Every one of these exercises has the advantage that the benefit is not too closely localized. Many other portions of the body receive benefit from the faithful performance of the feats that I have outlined for my reader.

The exercise shown by photographs 72 and 73 gives a very satisfactory task for the muscles that are employed in rotating the leg. From your reading of the preceding chapter you will remember just what muscles these are, and where they are located.

Now, with the help of my remarks in the last chapter, you can discover just what muscles you benefit by taking the exercise shown in the next two photographs. I am not going to help you out this time, as I have written enough concerning the muscles that are used in rising from a stooping position. Apply in the same manner what I have written and find out for yourself just what muscles are strengthened by the next exercise (see photographs 76 and 77).

Take a look at the photographs depicting the work

in exercise forty-three. Here the sartorius muscle is well employed. The other muscles that are also used thoroughly are indicated for you in the caption of photograph 81.

You remember, I hope, what I told you about the vastus externus muscle at the outer side of the leg. Study exercise forty-four and perform it then, and you will understand why I wish you to go through this feat frequently.

Then, for the muscles of the inner side of the upper leg, give a good trial to the exercise illustrated in photograph 82. Reverse the effect of this work by going through patiently with the feat shown in the next photograph (83).

Do not be in a hurry to get beyond the exercises that I have described so far. But, when you feel that you have secured a really good development of the muscles of the upper leg, and when you feel that you need harder work, you will find enough of it in the exercises depicted and explained in photographs 84 to 87.

In exercise forty-seven the important thing is to employ the muscles resistantly without anything outside pressing the leg. The idea is, when employing one set of muscles to bring the lower leg up, to press downward at the same time by the use of the opposing set of muscles. It is not usually easy to catch the resistant idea with full force during the first few trials, but after a little the knack comes to you. Be careful to employ enough resistance. This is decidedly strenuous work. Even a practiced athlete by putting in enough resistance, can tire his muscles after a little while.

Exercise forty-eight is still harder work if you do it with vim enough. Exercises forty-nine and fifty, as shown in photographs 86 and 87, can be made severe enough to quite lame you at first, if you repeat them more than a few times. But, as the muscles harden and grow in size, these exercises will become more and more like play.

Above all, in connection with these exercises, do not lose sight of the fact that you are doubling the value of the work if you do not fail to bear in mind just what muscles are affected. and *how* they are exercised. If you forget the uses of the muscles as I have explained them, turn back to the last chapter and study it again with care.

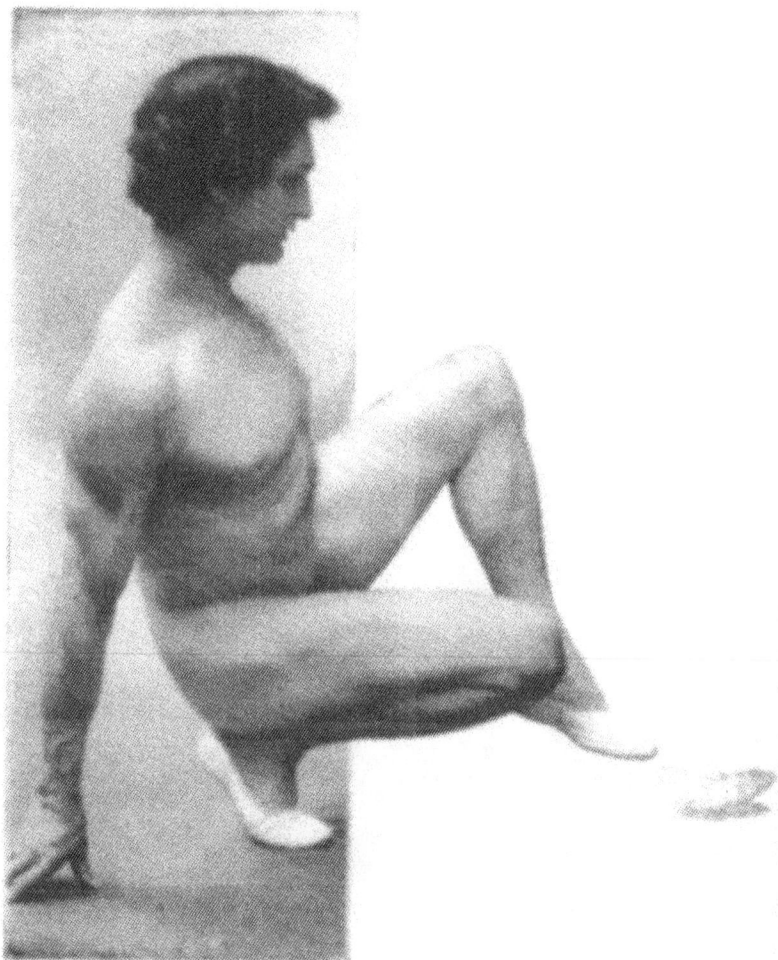

Photograph No. 71.

Exercise No. 39. Assume a squatting position, then balancing the body by placing the fingers of one hand on the floor, raise the left leg as high as you can. Same with the right leg. Continue the movement until the muscles tire. For strengthening muscles and tendons of abdomen, groin and extreme upper leg.

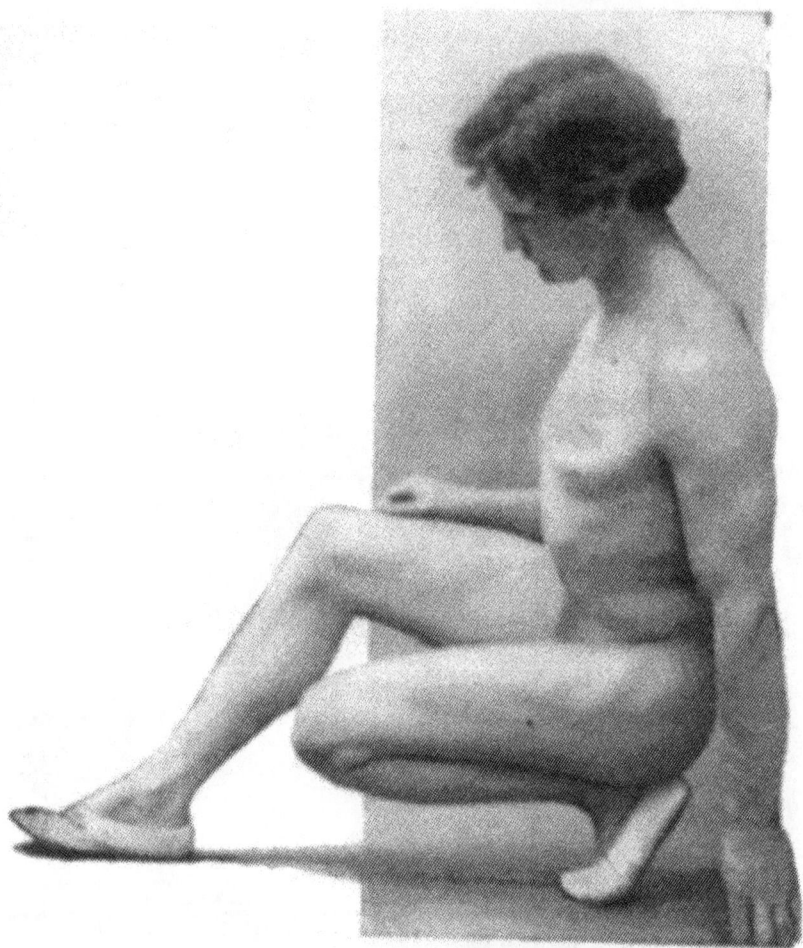

Photograph No. 72.

Exercise No. 40. Assume position shown in the photograph, balancing yourself by placing the fingers of the left hand on the floor. Now, without raising the body, turn the body slowly, and as you turn rest the weight on the right leg instead of the left (See next photo)

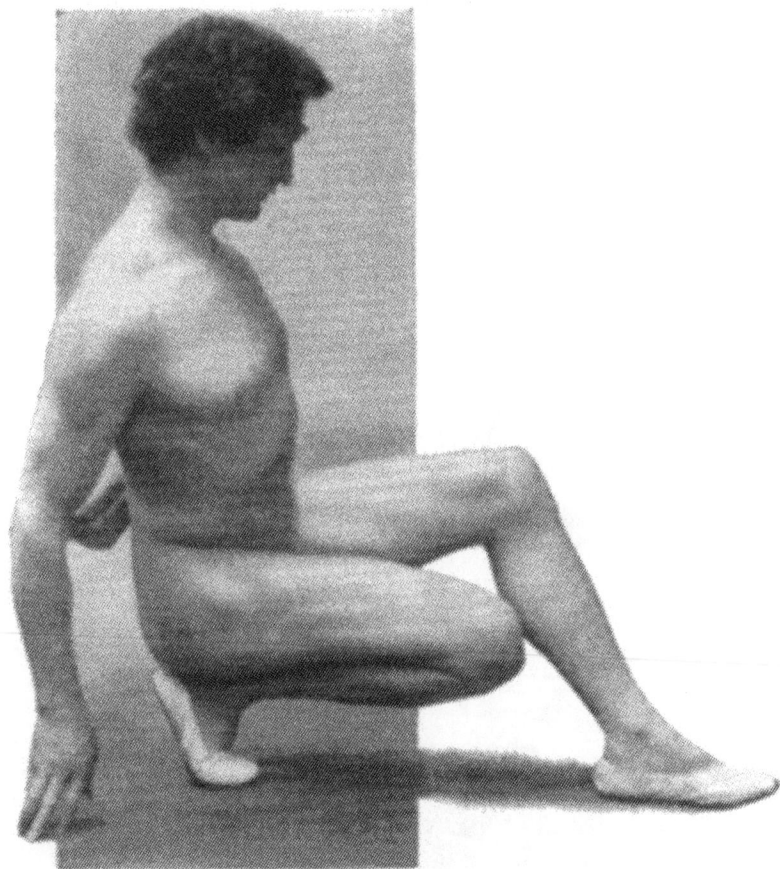

Photograph No. 73.

Until you assume the position as shown above, being exactly
similar to the preceding one, with the exception that the weight
is resting on the right leg instead of the left. Repeat the exercise until tired. When making this movement the foot is turned
on the floor with the weight resting thereon, and a pair of smooth
slippers or shoes will make the exercise more easy. This is
especially beneficial in rounding the knees and developing and
making more shapely the upper legs.

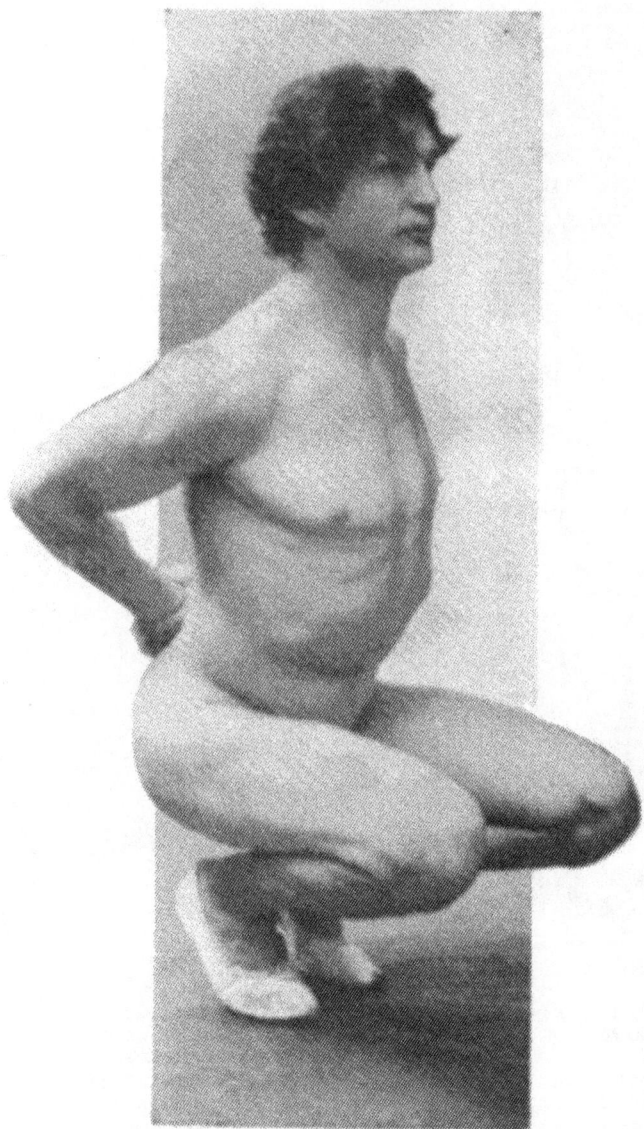

Photograph No. 74.

Exercise No. 41. Assume position as shown in illustration, with the hands clasped behind the back. Keep the body in a perpendicular position from the hips upward. Now rise (See next photo)

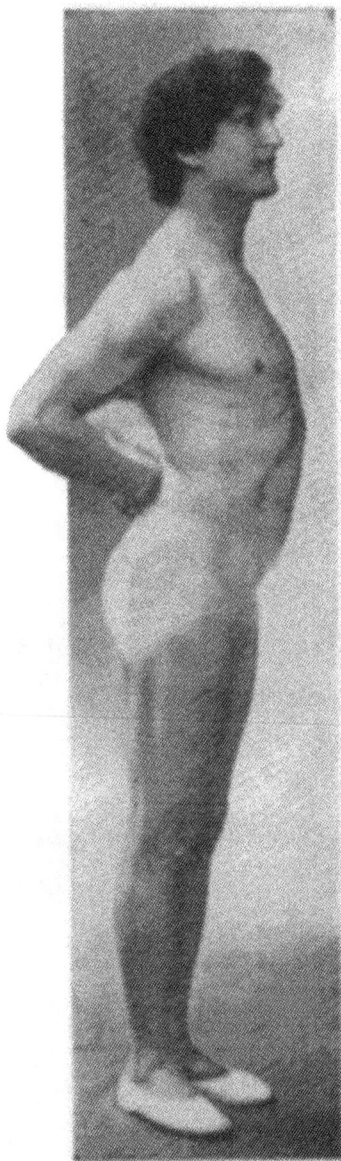

Photograph No. 75.

To above position. Repeat until tired. This is an old and simple exercise and is of great benefit for developing and strengthening the upper legs. The exercise can be taken quickly or slowly, as desired. It is better to vary the movements as to

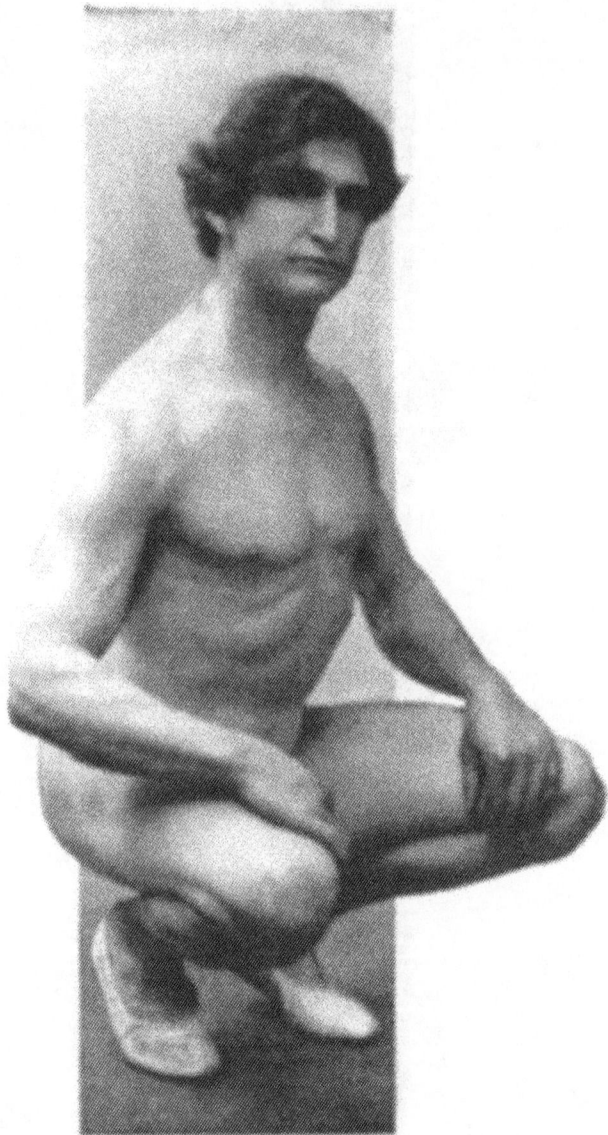

Photograph No. 76.

Exercise No. 42. Place the hands on the inside of the knees, as shown in illustration. If you cannot keep your balance in this position, lean against a chair or table. Now, resisting slightly with the hands, bring the knees inward until the hands touch (See next photo)

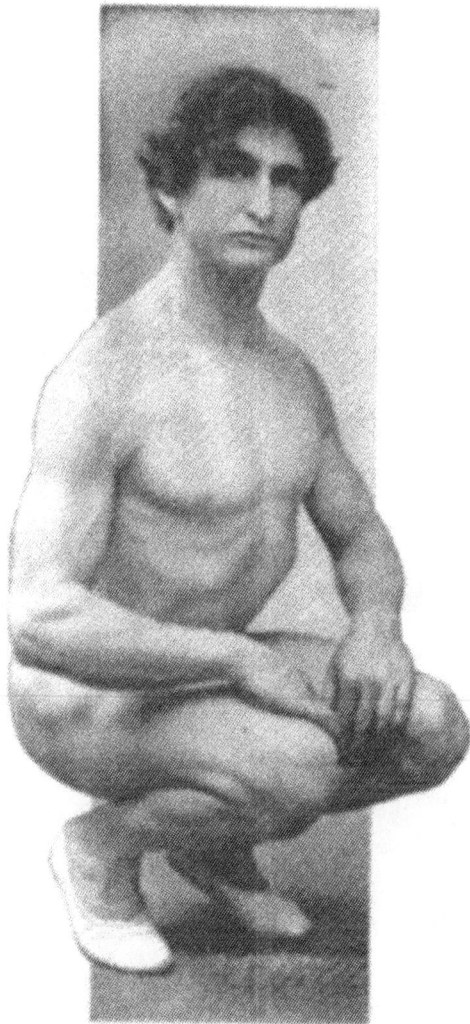

Photograph No. 77.

    As shown in above illustration. Repeat until tired. This exercise is especially valuable for developing the muscles on the inside of the upper thighs. These muscles give the upper leg a symmetrical contour and improve its appearance quite materially if properly developed. Many athletes with fairly well formed limbs have neglected to develop the muscles of this part of the leg, and naturally the leg does not appear symmetrically proportioned from all points of view. Horseback riding and all exercises that require an effort to bring the legs toward each other will assist in developing these muscles.

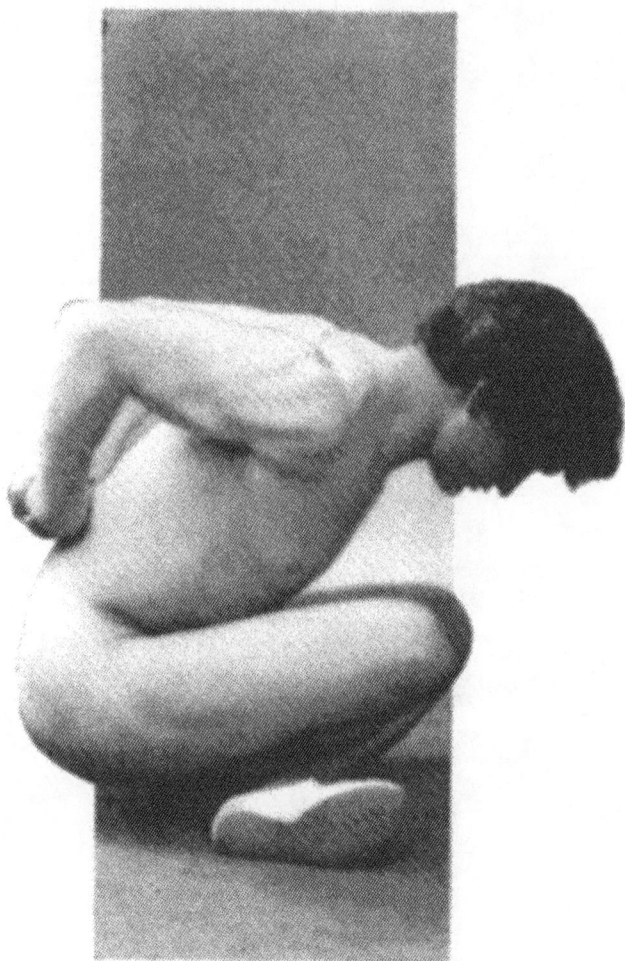

Photograph No. 78.

Exercise No. 43. Cross the legs tailor-fashion, clasping the hands behind the back, as shown in the illustration. If you find it difficult to assume this position, the easiest method will be to sit on the floor, then cross the calves of your legs under you, the left foot appearing under the right leg, and the right foot appearing under the left leg. Some prefer to begin the exercise standing, as shown in the next photograph. It does not make any particular difference which method is adopted, but after acquiring the position as shown above satisfactorily, rise slowly (See next photo)

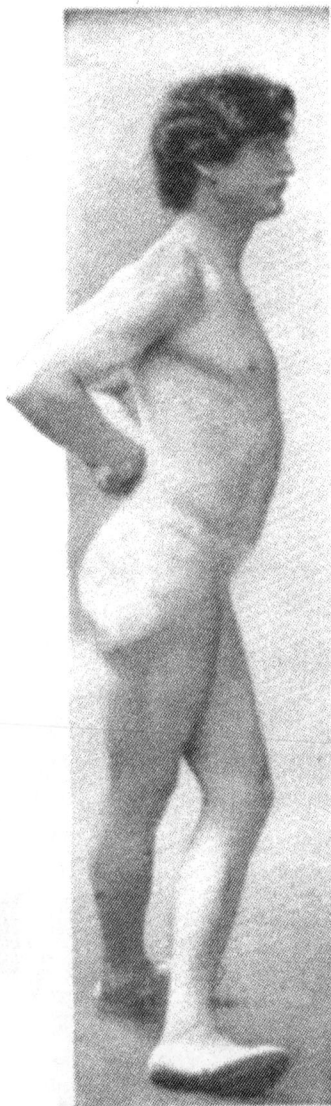

Photograph No. 79.

until in erect position as shown in this illustration. Return to the first position and continue the movement until tired. This exercise is especially beneficial for developing the muscles on the outside of the upper thighs and the central portions of the upper legs. It may be found difficult in the first few trials, though practice will enable you to perform it with ease. Should the exercises be found too difficult at first, start in the above position and bend the knees as far as will permit of your easily regaining a standing position.

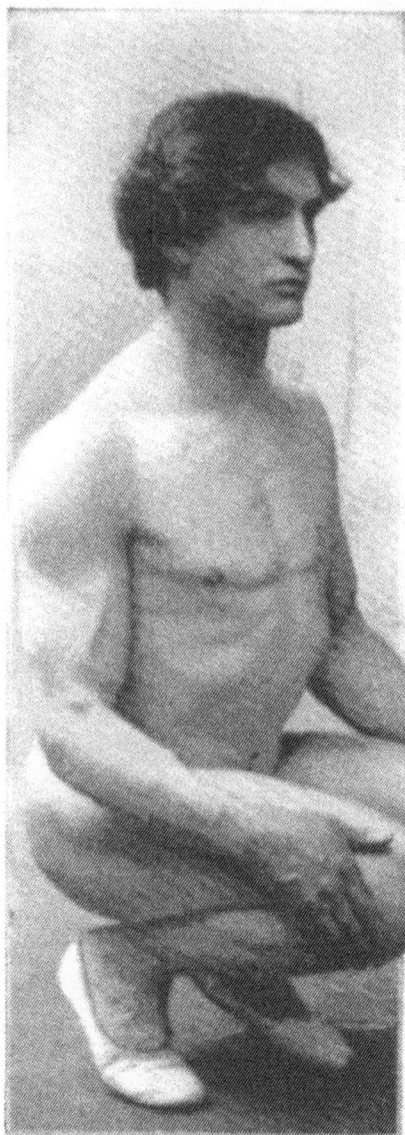

Photograph No. 86.

Exercise No. 44. Assume position shown in illustration, placing the hands on the outer side of each leg. While pressing inward with the hands, bring the legs outward (See next photo)

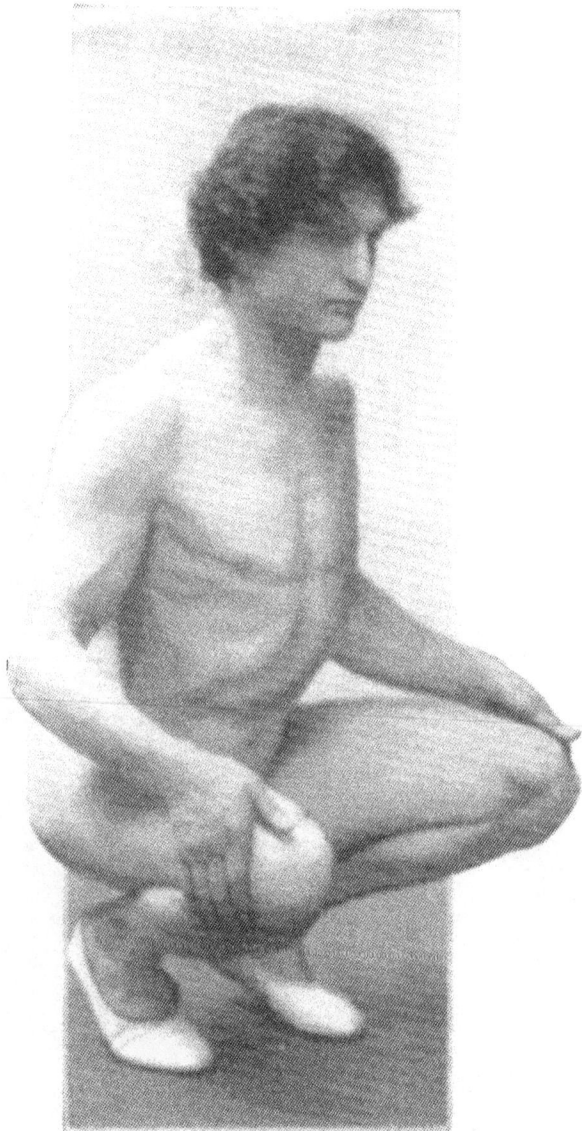

Photograph No. 81.

To position shown in above illustration. Continue the movement until the muscles tire. This exercise is especially good for developing the muscles of the outer side of the upper leg, though of course the crouching position tends to round the knees and develop all the muscles of the upper leg.

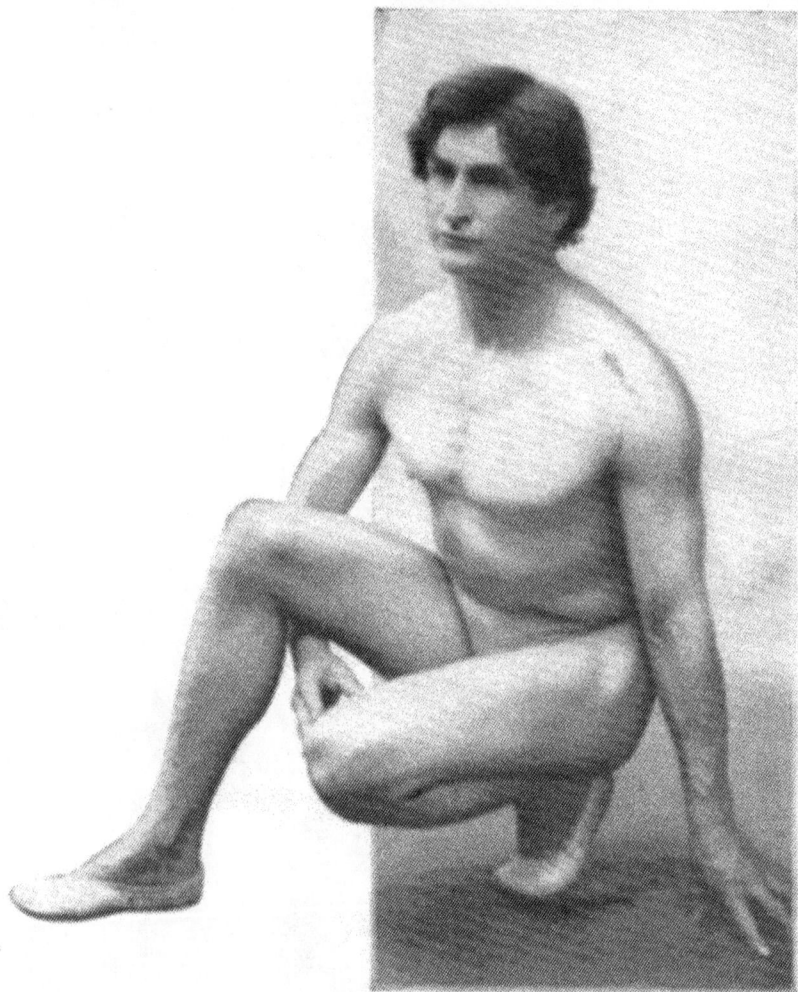

Photograph No. 82.

Exercise No. 45. Assume position shown in illustration. Place the fingers of the right hand on the inner side of the left knee as shown, then bring the left knee inward toward the right leg, pressing against the movement with the right hand. Continue the movement until the muscles tire. Same exercise with the position of the body reversed. This exercise is especially inclined to develop the muscles of the inner side of the upper leg.

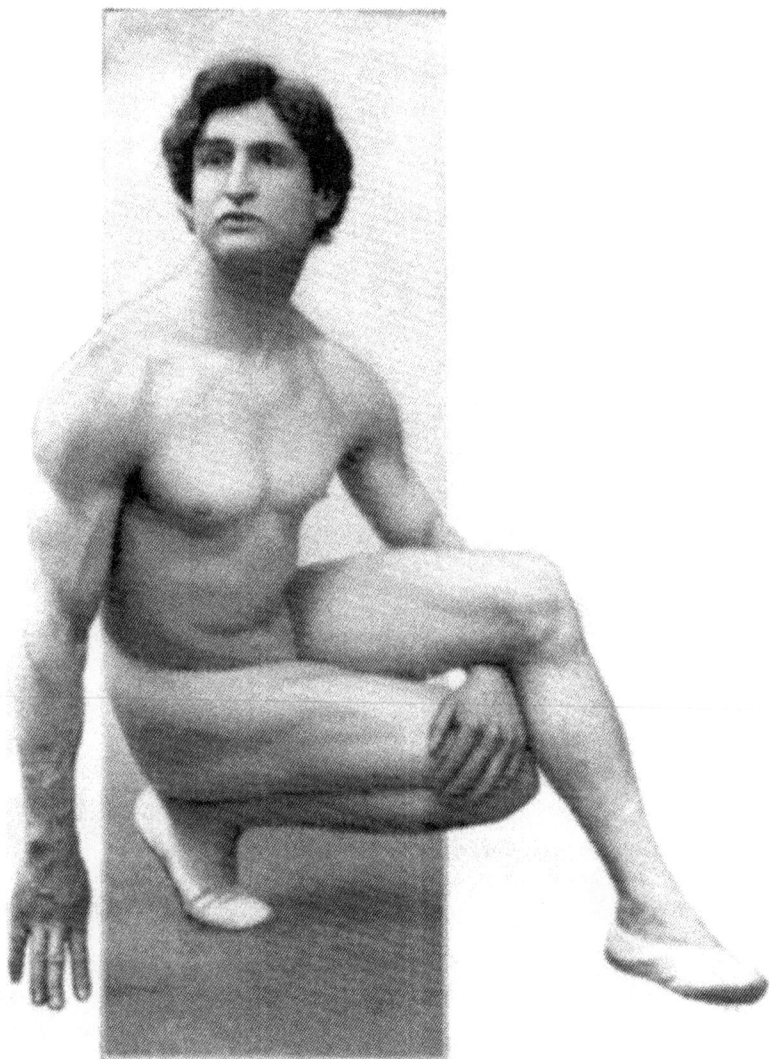

Photograph No. 83.

Exercise No. 46. Assume position shown in illustration, placing fingers on the floor to maintain balance. Clasp the outer side of the right leg with the left hand, then endeavor to bring the right leg outward away from the left leg as far as you can. Continue the movement until the muscles tire. Same exercise with position reversed. But little movement can be made in this exercise. It is a very good exercise to assist in developing the outer muscles of the upper thighs, and for general leg development.

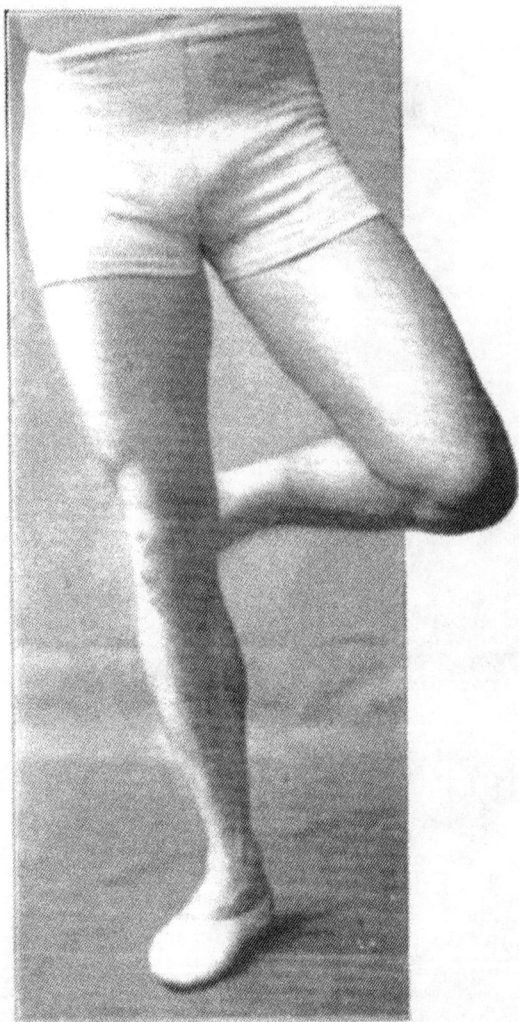

Photograph No. 84.

Exercise No. 47. Bend the left leg very slowly, bringing the foot upward as far as you can, tensing the muscles strongly while making the movement. In this exercise one muscle should resist the other, and you may not be able to make the movement correctly at the first attempt, but after a few trials you should perform it easily. Same exercise with the right leg. Continue movement of each leg until tired. For the muscles of the upper legs.

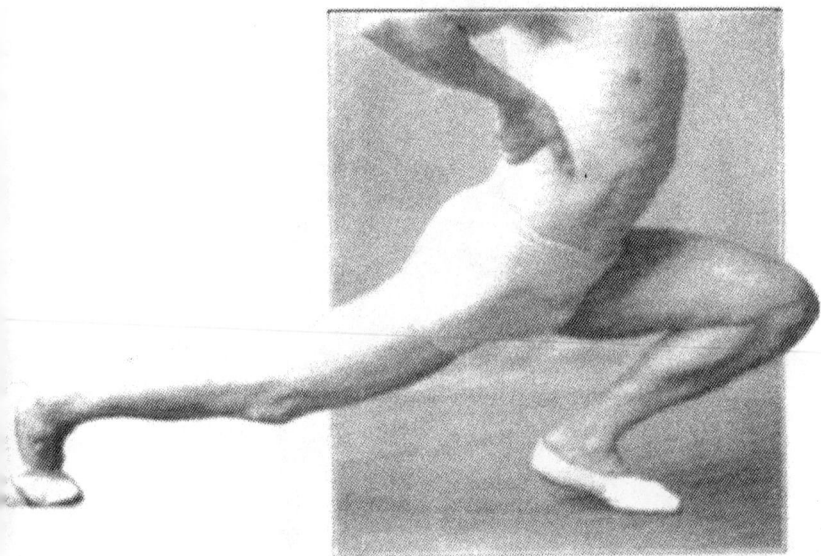

Photograph No. 85.

Exercise No. 48. Stand erect with left foot far forward. Now bend left leg as far as you can, as shown in above illustration. Straighten left leg and continue movement until slightly fatigued. Take the same exercise with the right leg forward. For muscles of the hip and upper leg.

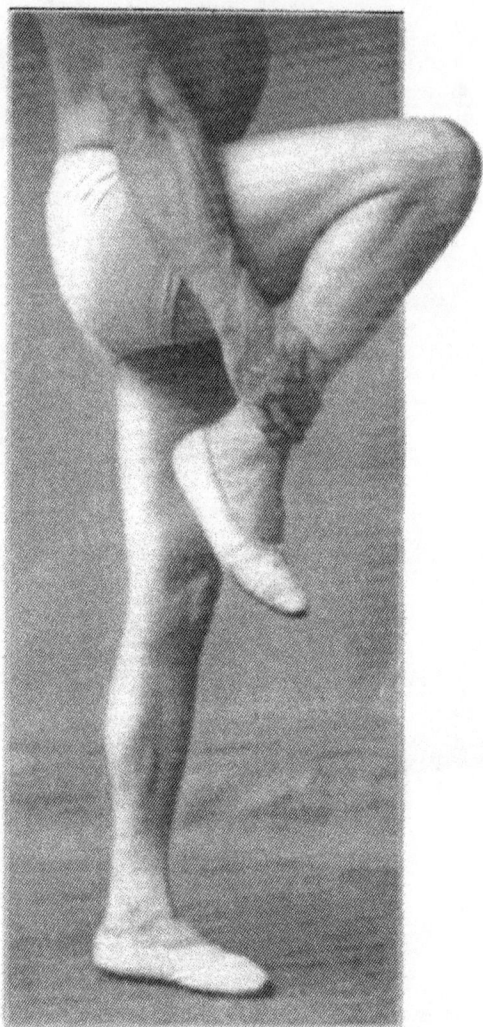

Photograph No. 86.

Exercise No. 49. Grasp ankle of right leg as shown in above illustration. Now straighten leg as far as you can, still maintaining your hold of the ankle. Back to original position and continue exercise until tired. Take same exercise with the left leg, grasping ankle with left hand. For muscles of upper leg.

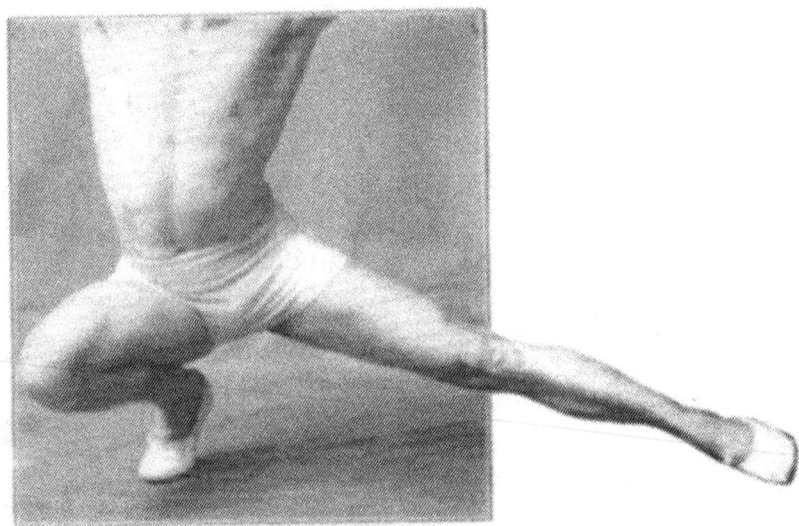

Photograph No. 87.

Exercise No. 50. Stand with feet far apart. Now slowly bend right knee and bring weight over to the right leg as shown in above illustration. When rising make the left leg assist as much as possible. Same exercise to the left. In this exercise the straight leg should be made to assist as much as possible each time you arise. If these instructions are followed this exercise uses very strongly the muscles on the inside of the upper leg.

CHAPTER XXIV.

Anatomical Structure of the Muscles of the Calves.

In this chapter I purpose to say something concerning the muscles at the front of the lower leg, but shall claim most of my reader's attention for a consideration of the muscles of the calf of the leg.

But, in the first place, let us understand the nature of the two bones that are to be found in the lower leg. Of these, the principal one is the tibia, which, in common parlance, we call the "shin bone." It articulates with the lower end of the thigh bone by means of what anatomists define as a "hinge joint."

The companion bone, the fibula—for which there is no common name—is of about the same length, but much more slender. It is found on the outer side of the leg, and is firmly joined to the tibia at either end. The lower end forms what we call commonly the outer ankle bone. The main purpose of the fibula is to assist in the various rotating movements of the leg, and also to aid the tibia in supporting the weight of the body and in the mechanism of walking.

Now the principal muscles in the front of the leg are known under the impressive names of the tibialis antious, the extensor proprius hallucis, the extensor longus digitorum and the peroneus tertius. There is a joke on the anatomists over the "hallucis" muscle. It refers to the great toe, but the word was invented by some anatomist whose knowledge of Latin was not as great as his zeal. The word should be "allicis." But by the time that the Latin scholars got after the anatomist the mischief was done, and the word "hallucis" had gotten into such general use that it remains in vogue to-day, and grave professors go on teaching the word "hallucis" when all the time they know that it should be "allicis." The word "hallucis" has been in use so long that no professor dares make the change to the right word, "allicis." This parallels some of the other traditions in medicine, which, right or wrong, must be preserved for the "honor of the profession."

The tibialis anticus is found on the outer side of the tibia. It is fleshy above, and all tendon below. Its task is to flex the sole of the foot, and to raise the inner border of the foot. The extensor proprius "hallucis" is the extensor muscle that affects the great toe. It is a long and flat muscle between the tibialis anticus and the extensor longus digitorum. And this latter muscle is also long and flat, and its function is to extend all the toes. The peroneus tertius is a part of the extensor longus digitorum, but its work is to flex the bones of the foot.

Now, dismissing these muscles of the front of the lower leg, we will pass on to the more important muscles of the calf. And first, we come to the gastrocnemius. This is the muscle nearest the surface in the back of the lower leg. It forms the greater part of the calf, and it is to the proper development of this muscle that the athlete must look for strength in the lower leg, while upon the perfection of this muscle depends also the shapeliness of the calf.

This muscle has two heads. The inner head is the larger, and arises near the base of the thigh bone. The

202 MUSCULAR POWER AND BEAUTY

outer and smaller head has its origin at the outside of
the lower end of the thigh bone and somewhat at the
back of the base of the thigh bone.

This muscle, for the main part, is a network of muscular fibres. At the lower end these fibres converge into
a tendinous form, and this combines with the tendon
of the soleus muscle to form the "tendon of Achilles."

More than passing attention should be paid to this
tendon of Achilles. It is the thickest and by long odds
the strongest tendon in the human body. It is some
six inches in length, beginning at about the middle of
the back of the lower leg. With the foot flexed it may
be felt very plainly just above the back of the heel.
Many people call it the "cord of the heel." The tendon
is a necessary part of the scheme of mechanism that
enables man to keep his upright position so easily.

The soleus is a broad, flat muscle that is found just
under the gastrocnemius, and is so called from its
resemblance to the shape of the fish named the sole.
The origin of this muscle is at the back part of the head
of the fibula and from the shaft of the same bone just
below; a further portion of the origin is also near the
head of the tibia. The fibres of the muscle form a
network at first, but gradually thicken and narrow
finally becoming the tendon that joins that of the
gastrocnemius to form the tendon of Achilles.

The third of the surface muscles of the calf that we
will consider, is the plantaris. As found in the human
leg this is a very small muscle that lies between the
gastrocnemius and the soleus. It is probably the rudi-
ment of a much larger muscle that existed in the human
body in past ages, for it is found strongly developed
in some of the lower animals. In the human body, the
fleshy portion of this muscle is only some three or four

inches in length, and it then becomes a slender tendor which is inserted into the tendon of Achilles at the heel.

The flexor muscles of the calf are found beneath those already described, forming the deep layer. This deep layer of muscles does not call for our consideration, for here, as in other parts of the body, the same work that brings superb development to the muscles near the surface, does the same for those of the deep layer.

We will return, therefore, to a consideration of the functions of the superficial muscles that I have already described. The work of the gastrocnemius muscle is to extend the foot. The soleus does the same work, although in a less degree, and with some difference of action. The plantaris aids both of the other muscles in extending the foot. Thus if you stand with one foot clear of the ground and point the toes downward, arching the foot, all three of the muscles are strained by the tension on them, and are relaxed when the foot is straightened again to its natural position. A very little thought, therefore, will show the student how important all of these muscles of the calf are in walking or running. Strength of these muscles, too, aids much in keeping one firmly in the stirrup when riding. The rower should have these muscles well developed, and is sure to improve them if he keeps steadily enough at his work with the oar. Conversely, faithful practice in the exercises that I shall describe in the next chapter, will prove a great aid to any athlete who wishes to prepare for walking, running, rowing, swimming and the other forms of work and sport that call for the best possible development of the calves.

Tests for gradual increase in the power of the muscles of the calf can be made in various ways. Perhaps the simplest and best method of making the test is to stand upon the toes with the heels clear of the ground, and to time the number of minutes and seconds that one is able to so stand without being obliged to let the heels down. A record showing the length of time that this test can be applied, from week to week, should furnish convincing testimony to the investigator as to whether he is growing stronger in these muscles.

Another very excellent way is to flex the foot strongly —that is, to bend the foot up toward the shin as much as possible, and while so doing feel the condition of the muscles in the calf with the hand.

Still another method is to be found by tensing the calf muscles strongly, and then slowly and *resistantly* rotating the foot in various ways. By "resistantly" I mean that every movement of rotation should be resisted by a tendency to use the opposing muscles in an effort to force the foot in the opposite direction. This rotating with resistance will throw out well developed calf muscles in very hard and prominent lumps of muscular fibre. It will show the investigator, also, just where the fleshy portions of the muscle in question are, where they cease and where the harder, firmer tendon begins.

It is well, also, to jot down the measurements of the calf at the very beginning of this development work, and to keep record of measurements taken every two or three weeks during the continuance of the exercising. Measurements will show that the development is slow, and at last a point will be reached where no amount of exercise of the muscles of the calf seems to greatly affect their proportions. By this time the athlete will have reached approximately the limit of development in the calf. If he is satisfied, at last, that this is really the case, the athlete will need the exercises for the calf muscles subsequently only in such a quantity as shall be sufficient to enable him to retain the benefit that he has gained.

But be careful never to lose sight of this maxim: *It is one thing to secure the proper development of the muscles in any portion of the body, and it is quite another thing to retain that development intact!*

Eternal vigilance is the price of the perfect body.

CHAPTER XXV.

Exercises for Developing the Muscles of the Calves.

Lest my reader imagine that I am over-zealous in presenting sixteen photographs illustrative of exercises for developing the muscles of the calves, I hasten to call his attention to the fact that the muscular effects of these exercises are not confined to the calves. Incidentally the whole leg is benefited by the work advised. The back muscles also come in for a very good share of work, and so do the abdominal muscles. The chest muscles get a little of the benefit as well, and the same is true of the neck muscles. Then too, the vital organs in the chest and abdomen have a certain amount of new vitality imparted to them. In fact, the arms and shoulders are the only portions of the body that do not benefit more or less from these exercises.

Exercise fifty-one (photographs 88 and 89) seems simple. A trial will convince you that there is plenty of hard and useful work in it. It paves the way, too, for one of the tests that I mentioned in the last chapter. This is what might be called the fundamental feat in the development of splendid muscles in the calves.

Exercise fifty-two is a reversal of 51, but reversals have a value of their own in calling for an exactly opposite change in the employment of the muscles. Exercise fifty-four offers a distinct change in the line of work, but exercise fifty-five carries us back again to the use of the block of wood.

Give more than the usual amount of attention to the practice of exercise fifty-six. At first a tedious feat, it gives a strength to the calf muscles that is sure to delight him who wishes to go in strongly for walking and running. This feat should be a favorite with all enthusiastic track workers.

There is much fatigue in store for the beginner who takes up exercise fifty-seven, but it should be persevered in. It gives rather severe employment to the muscles at the sides of the calf, and with corresponding benefit in increased strength there. This, too, is work that is especially advisable for the lover of the track. Exercise fifty-eight supplies the necessary reversal of the work.

Photograph 98 gives the idea of exercise fifty-nine, but there is one point of this feat that no illustration can cover. That is the intensity of the resistance to be supplied by the fingers against the outward progress of the toes. This resistance should be made just as hard as the movement of the feet can overcome.

The same remark applies to exercise sixty. In exercise sixty-one, the style of resistance is changed completely, and comes from the weight of the body, alternately on the toes and on the heels. This last exercise, if performed with sufficient speed, makes greatly both for agility of the legs and for balance upon them. It is excellent practice for the calves in some of the most representative movements that they can be called upon to perform.

Observe exercise sixty-two, as shown in photograph 101. Look at the illustration closely and see how prominently the gastrocnemius muscle appears. In the left leg you will note the termination of the fleshy "belly" of the muscle, and at that point the tendon begins which becomes a part of the tendon of Achilles to which I made allusion in the last chapter.

The last exercise, sixty-three, calls for work that would be severe upon a beginner if carried out with zeal.   But he who has been persistently using the other exercises for the calf muscles for a few days, should find this exercise a simple and easy one now.

"Practice makes perfect."   But in exercising in the right way, persistent practice does more—it supplies new strength with which to combat threatened fatigue.

There are some who claim to experience the greatest difficulty in developing their calves, for while they have perhaps practiced physical culture for a considerable length of time, and may really enjoy vigorous health and a satisfactory degree of all around strength, yet they are not satisfied with the size of these particular parts.   For such as these, especially, I would suggest the most persistent and faithful application to the exercises illustrated in connection with this chapter. It will probably require some degree of determination to keep you at it, but if you are willing to devote yourself earnestly to them for a sufficient length of time, the results are absolutely certain.   That is to say, you will surely reach the limit of your natural development.

There are several other means of improving the size of the calf which are often convenient and which in such cases are valuable as helping somewhat to secure the final result, for instance, hill climbing, especially long and steep hills.   In climbing either hills or stairways, it is important that you endeavor to make the calves do most of the work, rising high on the toes with each step. As a matter of fact, you will find that you can climb difficult hills far more easily by this method than by walking on the heels, in which case the upper leg is forced to do most of the work. By means of this natural use of the muscles of the calf, you will find that you can negotiate a long hill or a series of stairs in a building of many stories with little or none of that sense of general bodily fatigue or exhaustion which is common, even though your efforts may have succeeded in making the calves themselves ache.

Rising high on the toes while lifting and holding very heavy weights is also conducive to a rapid development of the parts in question, though not favorable to endurance, speed and elasticity of the muscles affected. However, neither this nor the practice of hill climbing, though of course helpful, will offer you as sufficient a means of calf development as the exercises illustrated herewith.

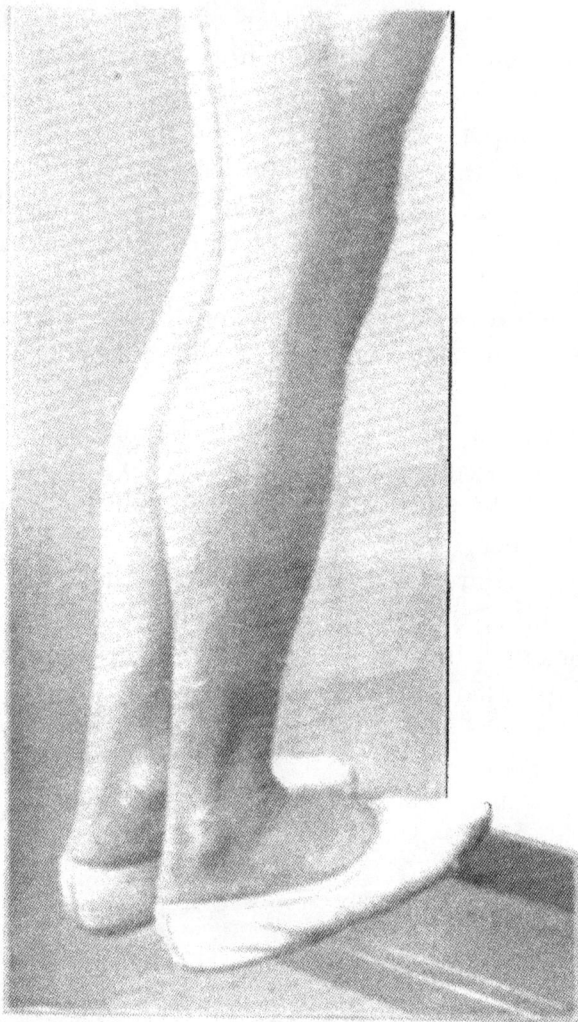

Photograph No. 88.

Exercise No. 51. Secure a piece of wood of some kind that will raise you about four inches from the floor. Stand on the extreme edge of this with the toes as shown in illustration, allowing the body to sink as far as you can. Now rise slowly. (See next photo.)

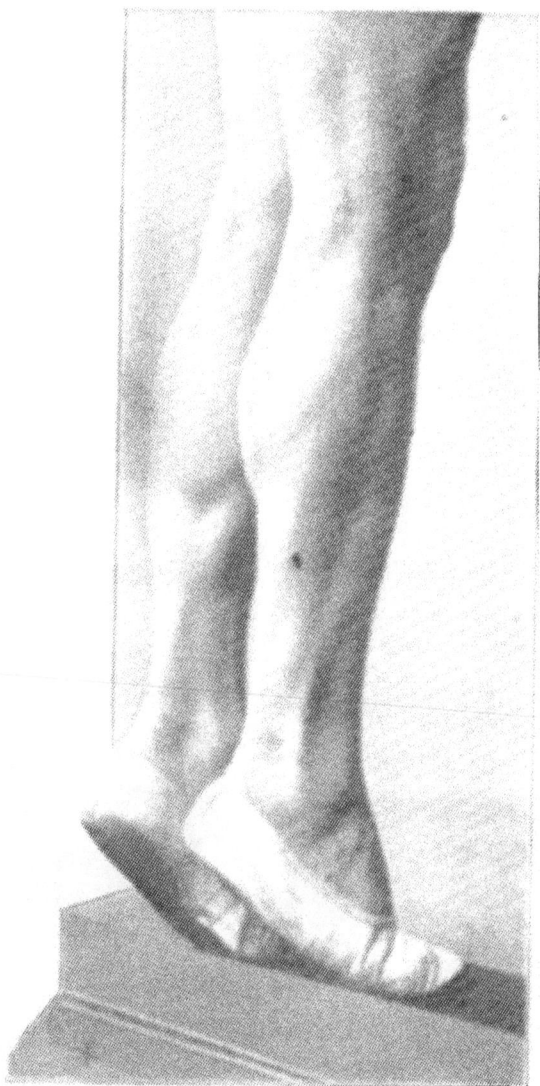

Photograph No. 89.

As high as you can, as shown in above illustration. Sink back into former position and continue until muscles tire. This is another very strenuous exercise for the large muscles on the back of the calf.

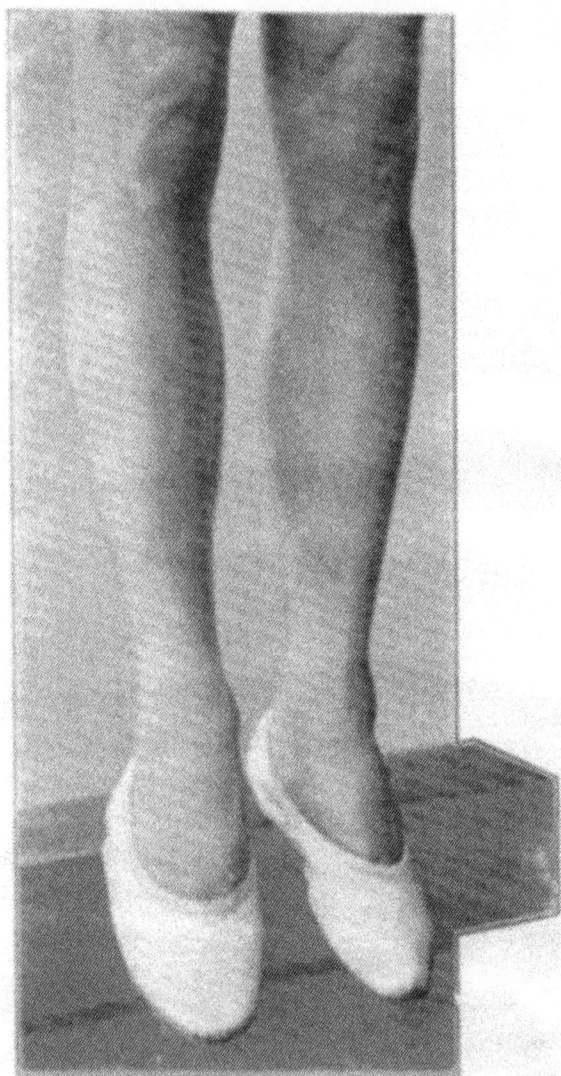

Photograph No. 90.

Exercise No. 52. Stand on the block of wood described previously, with the heels as shown in the illustration, reaching downward with the toes as far as you can. Now raise the toes (See next photo)

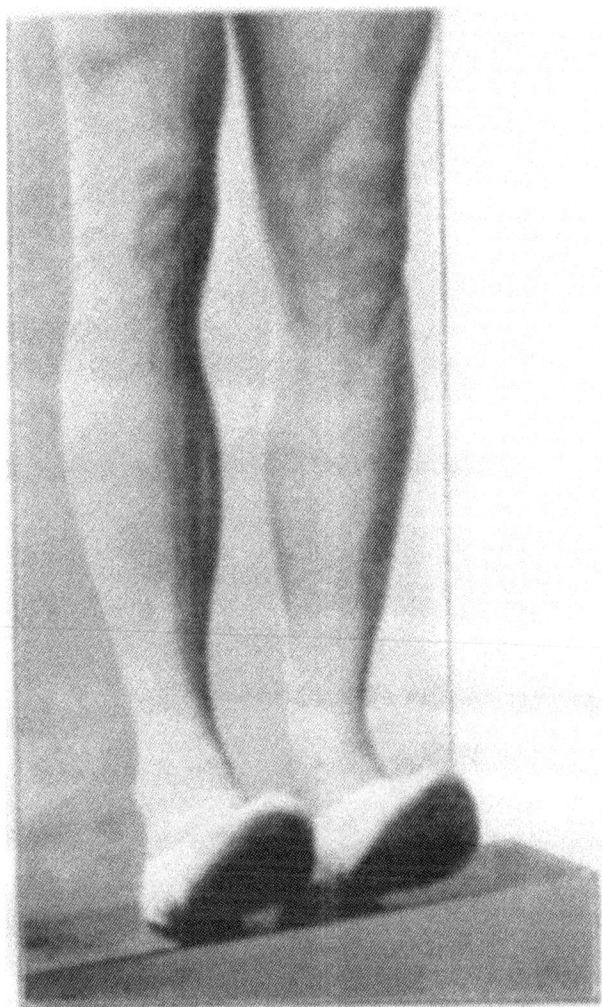

Photograph No. 91.

As high as you can, as shown in above illustration. Repeat movement until tired. This is superior exercise for developing the flat muscles on the front of the calf.

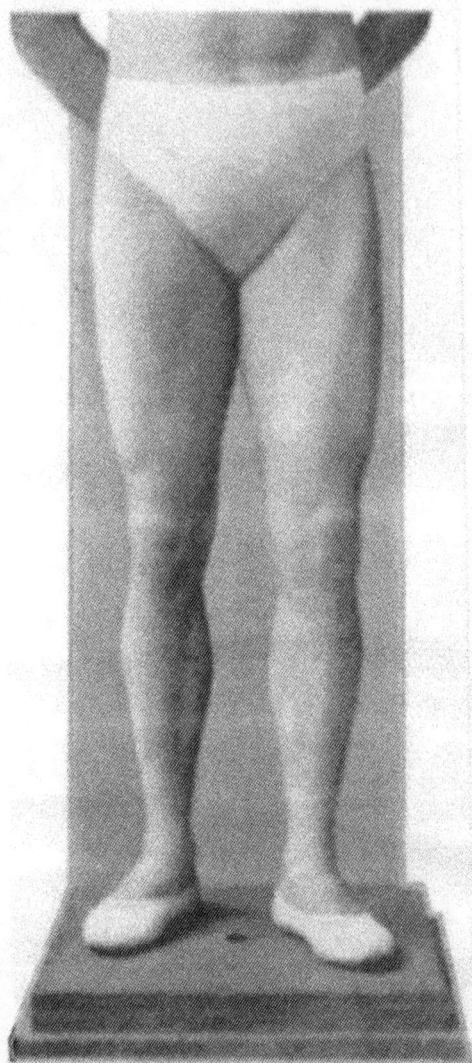

Photograph No. 92.

Exercise No. 53. Stand with one foot slightly in front of the other. Now rise on the toes as high as you can, then, remaining in this position, make several attempts to rise still higher on the toes. Repeat with the right and left foot forward alternately until tired. This is a very vigorous exercise for the large muscle on the back of the calf.

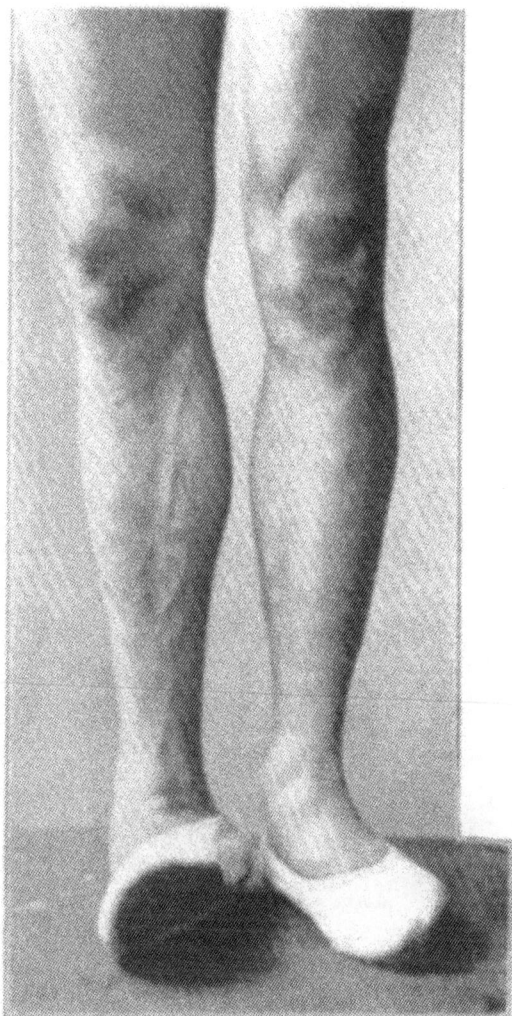

Photograph No. 93.

Exercise No. 54. Stand flat on both feet. Now twist the body slightly, allowing the ankles to turn until the weight is resting on the outside of the right foot and the inside of the left foot. Then twist in the opposite direction, reversing the position. Continue movement until muscles tire. This is a splendid exercise for strengthening the ankles and the muscles on the inside and outside of the calves.

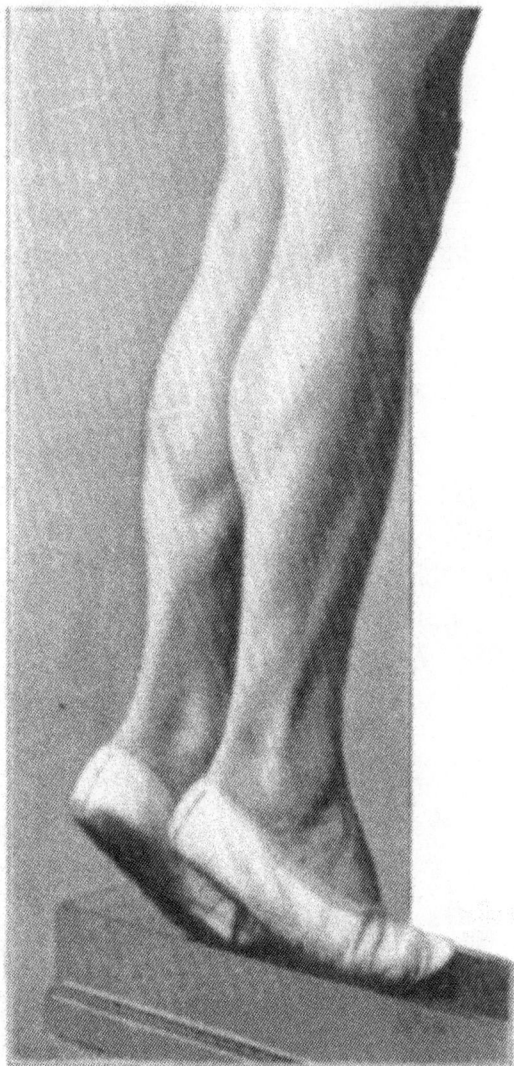

Photograph No. 94.

Exercise No. 55. Rise as high as you can on toes as shown in illustration. Now, maintaining this position, turn the feet so the weight will rest mostly on the outer edge of the toes. Then turn back and rest the weight as nearly as you can on the large toes. Continue this exercise, rolling back and forth, until the muscles tire. For the muscles on the outside and the inside of the calf.

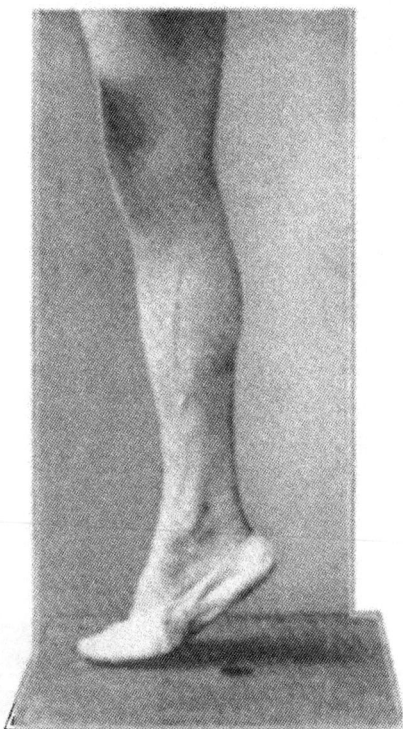

Photograph No. 95.

Exercise No. 56. Stand with the weight on one foot and rise on the toes as high as you can, as shown in illustration. After tiring the muscles of one leg repeat the exercise with the weight resting on the other foot. For the muscles on the back of the calf.

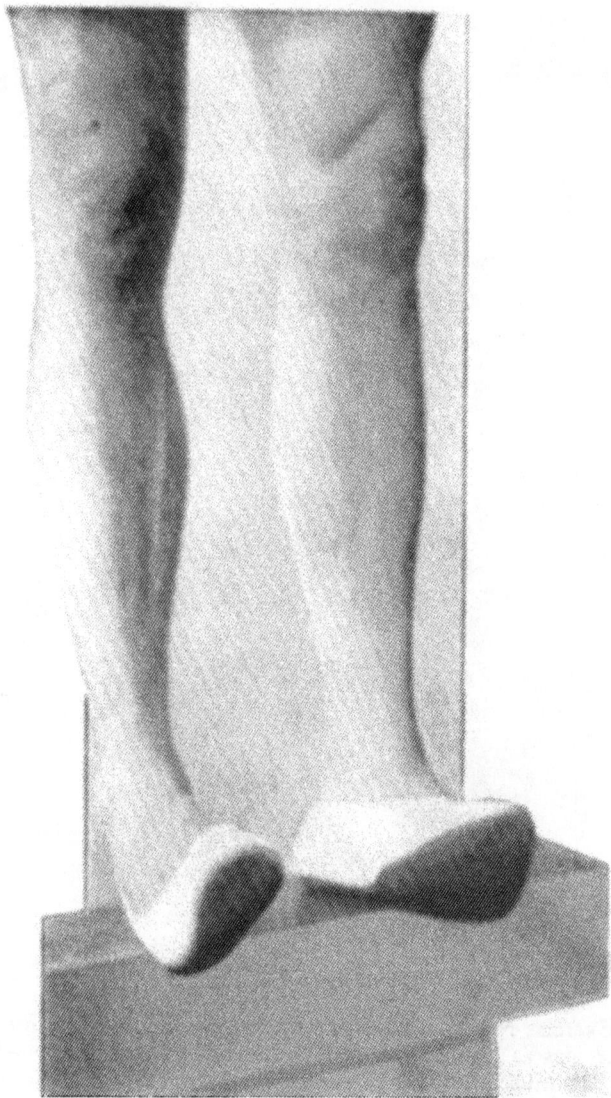

Photograph No 96.

Exercise No. 57. Stand on the heels, on the edge of a block of wood, as shown. Now, bend the ankles and roll the foot outward until the weight rests on the outer sides of the feet, and roll them in the other direction until the weight rests on the inner sides of the feet. Continue the exercise back and forth until the muscles tire. For the muscles on the inner and outer sides of the calf.

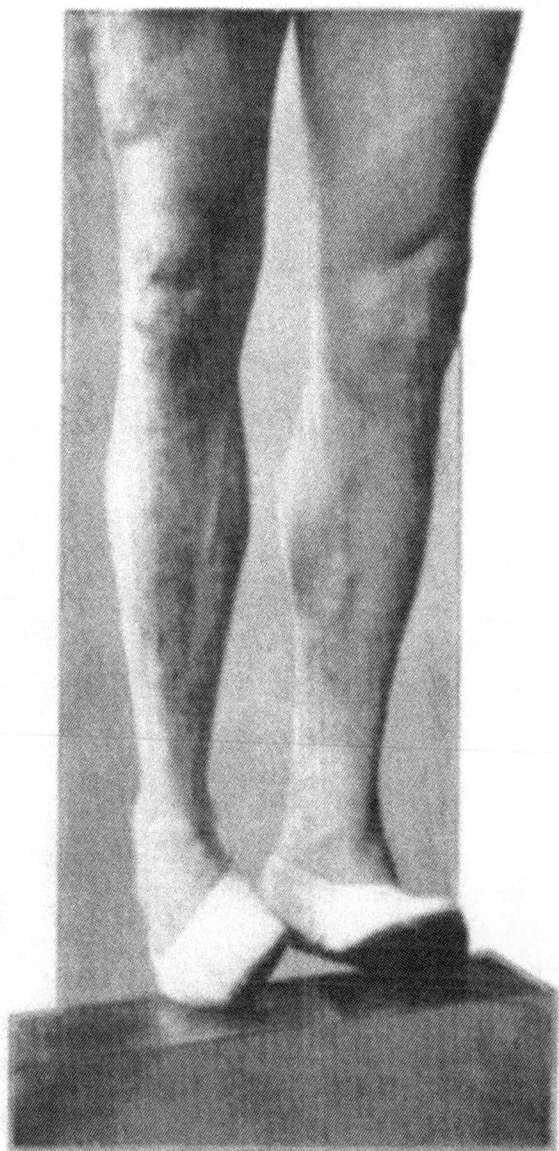

Photograph No. 97.

Exercise No. 58. Stand with the toes resting on the block of wood or the edge of a stair. Roll the feet until the weight of the body is resting on the outer sides of the feet. Then roll the feet in the opposite direction until the weight is resting on the inner sides of the feet. Continue exercise back and forth until tired. For the muscles on the inner and outer sides of the calf.

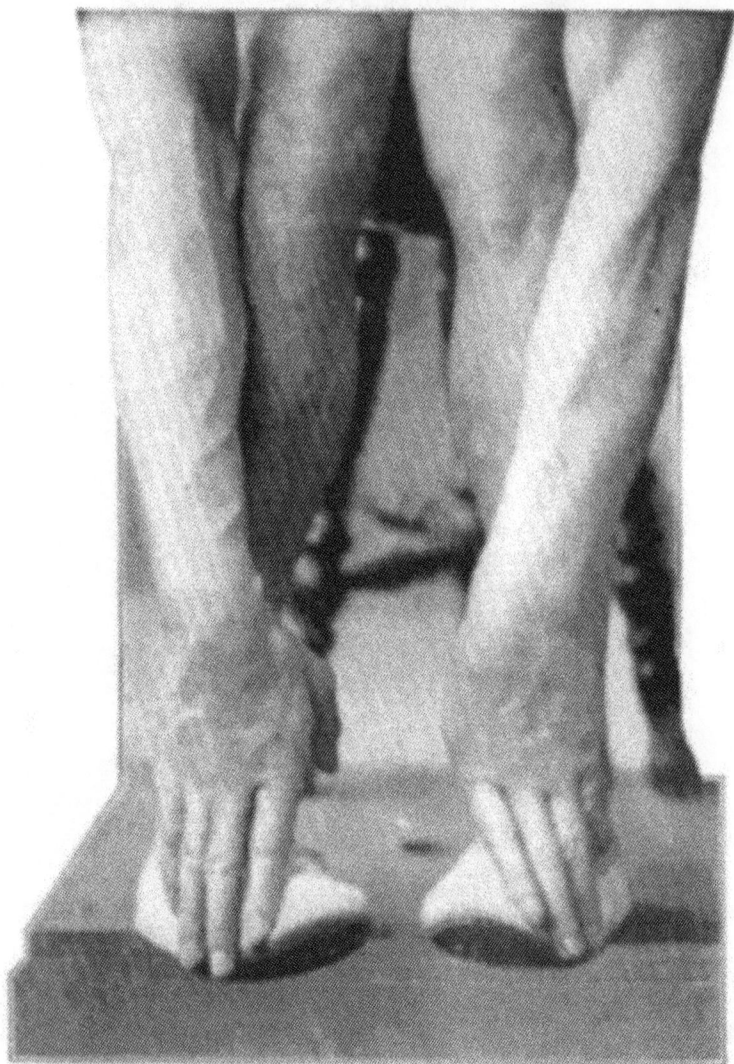

Photograph No. 98.

Exercise No. 59. Seat yourself on a chair. Now, reach down and place your hands on the outer sides of the toes, as shown in the illustration. Now, bring the toes outward as far as you can, pressing against the movement slightly with the fingers of the hand. Continue the exercise back and forth until tired. For the twisting muscles of the calves and upper legs.

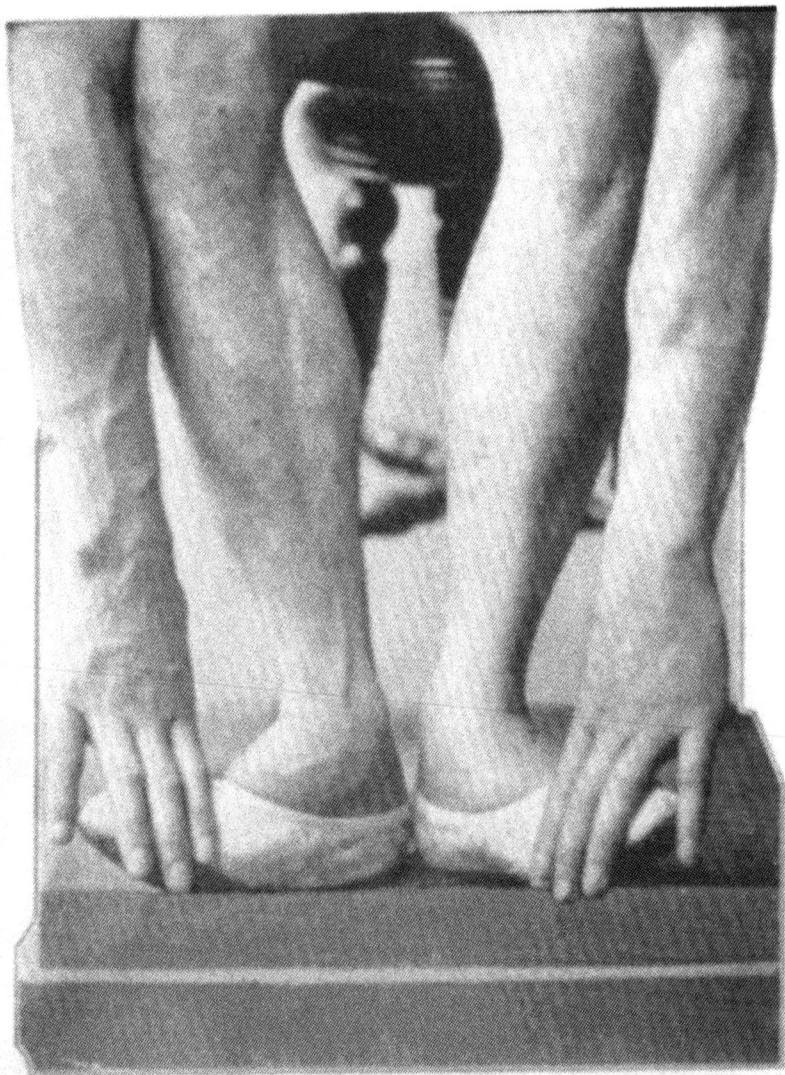

Photograph No. 99.

Exercise No. 60. Seat yourself on a chair and place hands on the inner sides of the feet while turned far outward as shown in illustration. Now, bring the toes of the feet together, pressing slightly against the motion with the fingers. Continue until tired. For the twisting muscles of the calves and legs and upper legs.

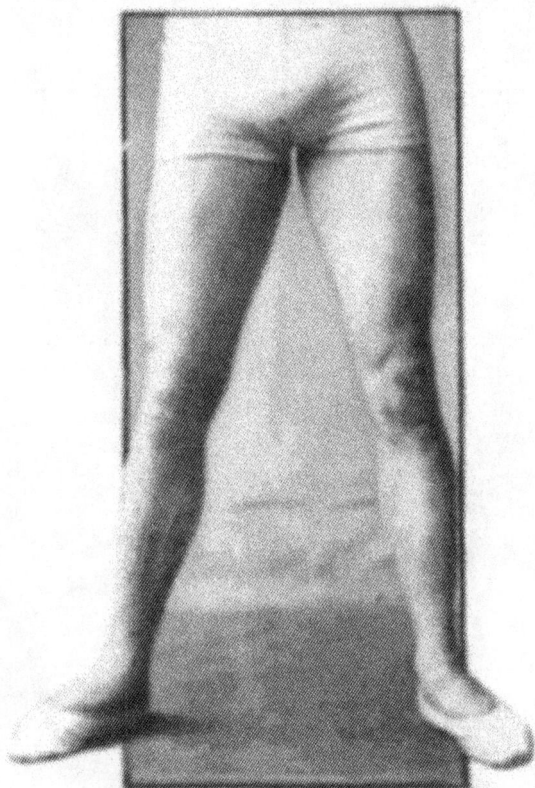

Photograph No. 100.

Exercise No. 61. Stand with the feet in position snown above. Bear the weight of the body on the heels and turn the toes outward as far as you can. Now change the weight to the toes and move the heels outward as far as possible. Continue this exercise until the legs are as far out as they will go without pain. Reverse the exercise, bringing the feet slowly together. Continue back and forth until the muscles tire.

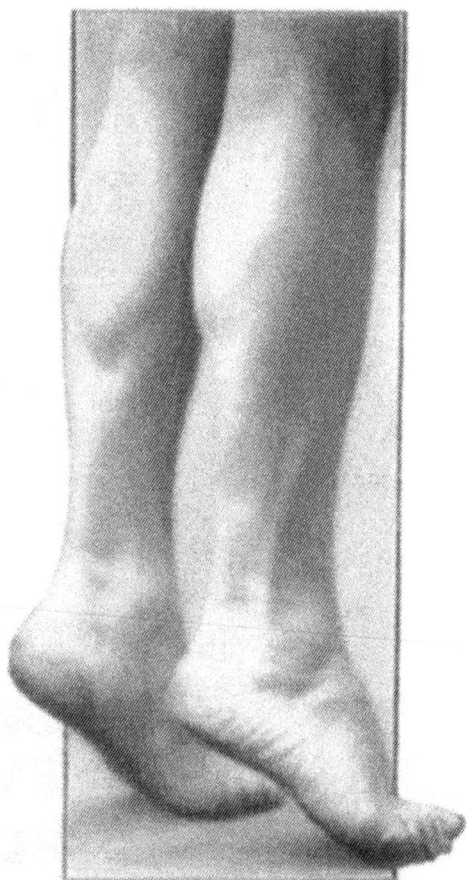

Photograph No. 101.

Exercise No. 62. Rise on toes as high as you can, as shown in illustration. Now, maintaining this position, make an effort to rise still higher. Repeat this until the muscles are slightly tired. It is an especially valuable exercise for developing the muscles on the back of the calves.

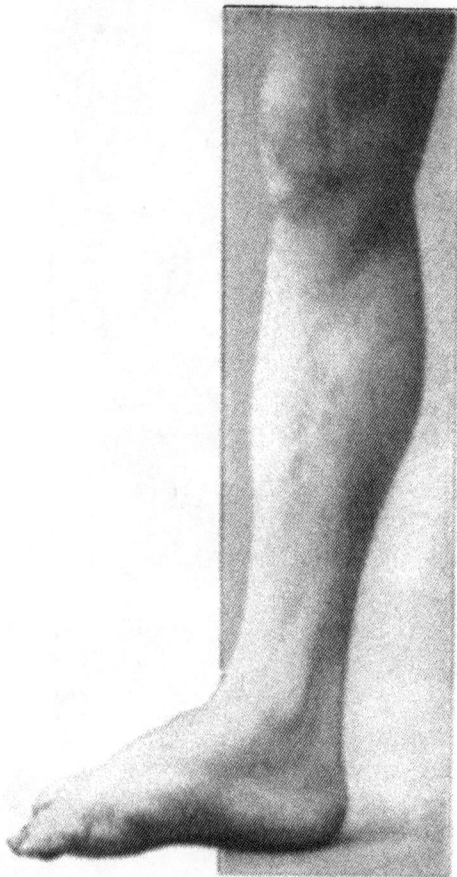

Photograph No. 102.

Exercise No. 63. Raising the right foot free from the floor,
reach with the toes downward as far as you can, as illustrated
Now, raise the toe upward (See next photo)

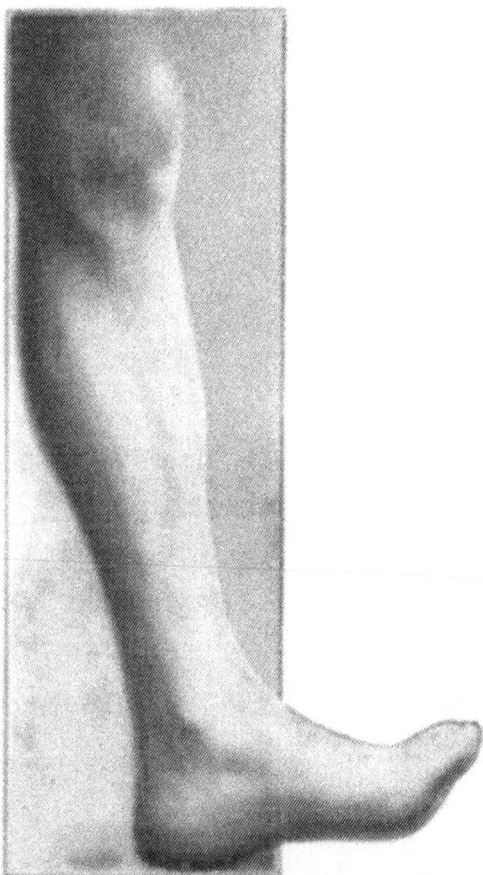

Photograph No. 103.

As far as you can, as shown in above illustration.   Continue movement until tired.   For developing the small muscles on the front part of the calf.

www.ingramcontent.com/pod-product-compliance
Lightning Source LLC
Chambersburg PA
CBHW020609270326
41927CB00005B/246